General
Practice

(CLINICAL CASES UNCOVERED)

KT-492-869

BMA LIBRARY
BRITISH MEDICAL ASSOCIATION

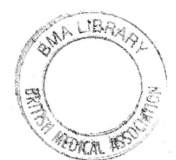

WITHDRAWN FROM LIBRARY

BRITISH MEDICAL ASSOCIATION

0761606

BMA

1

BMA Library

Freepost RTKJ-RKSZ-JGHG
British Medical Association
PO Box 291
LONDON
WC1H 9TG

FREE RETURN POSTAGE FOR STUDENTS & FY DOCTORS!

Use this label for the **FREE** return of books to the BMA Library

General Practice

CLINICAL CASES UNCOVERED

Emma Storr

BA (Hons), MRCGP, DRCOG,
PG Cert (LTHE)

Senior Clinical Lecturer
Department of General Practice
Dunedin School of Medicine
University of Otago
New Zealand

Alison Lea

BSc (Hons), MBChB, MRCGP,
PG Cert (PCE)

Senior Clinical Teaching Fellow
Academic Unit of Primary Care
Leeds Institute of Health Sciences
University of Leeds
Leeds

Sheena McMain

MBChB, MRCP, FRCGP,
MMedSci (PHC)

Associate Director General Practice
Yorkshire Deanery
University of Leeds
Leeds

Gail Nicholls

BSc, MBChB, MRCGP,
PG Cert (PCE)

Senior Clinical Teaching Fellow
Academic Unit of Primary Care
Leeds Institute of Health Sciences
University of Leeds
Leeds

Martha Leigh

BA (Hons), MBBS, DRCOG, DCH

GP Principal
Wapping Health Centre
London

⟨W⟩ WILEY-BLACKWELL

A John Wiley & Sons, Ltd., Publication

This edition first published 2008, © 2008 by E. Storr, G. Nicholls A. Lea, M. Leigh, S. McMain

Blackwell Publishing was acquired by John Wiley & Sons in February 2007. Blackwell's publishing program has been merged with Wiley's global Scientific, Technical and Medical business to form Wiley-Blackwell.

Registered office: John Wiley & Sons Ltd, The Atrium, Southern Gate, Chichester, West Sussex, PO19 8SQ, UK

Editorial offices: 9600 Garsington Road, Oxford, OX4 2DQ, UK
                        The Atrium, Southern Gate, Chichester, West Sussex, PO19 8SQ, UK
                        111 River Street, Hoboken, NJ 07030-5774, USA

For details of our global editorial offices, for customer services and for information about how to apply for permission to reuse the copyright material in this book please see our website at www.wiley.com/wiley-blackwell

The right of the author to be identified as the author of this work has been asserted in accordance with the Copyright, Designs and Patents Act 1988.

All rights reserved. No part of this publication may be reproduced, stored in a retrieval system, or transmitted, in any form or by any means, electronic, mechanical, photocopying, recording or otherwise, except as permitted by the UK Copyright, Designs and Patents Act 1988, without the permission of the publisher.

Wiley also publishes its books in a variety of electronic formats. Some content that appears in print may not be available in electronic books.

Designations used by companies to distinguish their products are often claimed as trademarks. All brand names and product names used in this book are trade names, service marks, trademarks or registered trademarks of their respective owners. The publisher is not associated with any product or vendor mentioned in this book. This publication is designed to provide accurate and authoritative information in regard to the subject matter covered. It is sold on the understanding that the publisher is not engaged in rendering professional services. If professional advice or other expert assistance is required, the services of a competent professional should be sought.

Library of Congress Cataloguing-in-Publication Data

General practice : clinical cases uncovered / Emma Storr . . . [et al.].
        p. ; cm.
   Includes bibliographical references and indexes.
   ISBN 978-1-4051-6140-4 (alk. paper)
   1.   Family medicine–Case studies.   2.   Internal medicine–Case studies.   I.   Storr, Emma.
   [DNLM: 1.   Family Practice–Case Reports.   WB 110 G3265 2008]
   RC66.G46 2008
   616–dc22

                                                                            2008003443

ISBN: 978-1-4051-6140-4

A catalogue record for this book is available from the British Library

Set in 9/12pt Minion by SNP Best-set Typesetter Ltd., Hong Kong

3   2010

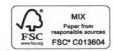

Contents

Colour plate section can be found between pp. 56–57.

Preface

We wrote this book to encourage individuals to learn about general practice in a challenging and stimulating way. Collectively, we have many years experience in the specialty and understand the complexity involved in dealing with patients in the community. People often do not fit the textbook descriptions of disease, and management of their clinical problems is a constant challenge. Our aim is to introduce 'real life' characters, with an array of medical, psychological and social problems. Not every case has a final or happy resolution, which reflects the reality of dealing with individuals with multiple concerns and varying medical conditions.

The book is organized into 36 cases which represent many of the common problems that GPs see. You will notice different styles and approaches in the writing, reflecting the authors' personalities, as well as the variety of patients who turn up at the surgery. We are well aware that due to lack of space and time, some patient scenarios are missing, including those which involve severe psychiatric problems and people with special needs. Despite that, we think the individuals presented here illustrate many of the types of people and conditions that GPs deal with on an everyday basis.

As each patient story progresses, new information or questions are presented that invite the student to solve the problem, make a differential diagnosis and think what they would do next. The reader's clinical knowledge and judgement are tested, as well as their common sense. The case summary and key points section discuss the latest evidence and point to further reading. A self-assessment section relating to the cases is included at the end of the book to reinforce the factual information presented.

This book is aimed at senior medical students and junior doctors who are entering general practice as part of their training. We hope they will enjoy this book as an introduction to the huge variety of patients they will see in the community and appreciate the holistic approach taken by GPs, which is reflected in the text.

We would like to thank all our patients and colleagues who enabled us to gain unique experience and enjoy the challenge of practicing the 'art of medicine' in the general practice setting.

Emma Storr
Gail Nicholls
Alison Lea
Martha Leigh
Sheena McMain
2008

How to use this book

Clinical Cases Uncovered (CCU) books are carefully designed to help supplement your clinical experience and assist with refreshing your memory when revising. Each book is divided into three sections: Part 1, Basics; Part 2, Cases; and Part 3, Self-assessment.

Part 1 gives a quick reminder of the basic science, history and examination, and key diagnoses in the area. Part 2 contains many of the clinical presentations you would expect to see on the wards or crop up in exams, with questions and answers leading you through each case. New information, such as test results, is revealed as events unfold and each case concludes with a handy case summary explaining the key points. Part 3 allows you to test your learning with several question styles (MCQs, EMQs and SAQs), each with a strong clinical focus.

Whether reading individually or working as part of a group, we hope you will enjoy using your CCU book. If you have any recommendations on how we could improve the series, please do let us know by contacting us at: medstudentuk@oxon.blackwellpublishing.com.

Disclaimer

CCU patients are designed to reflect real life, with their own reports of symptoms and concerns. Please note that all names used are entirely fictitious and any similarity to patients, alive or dead, is coincidental.

Setting the context

The art of general practice

The practice of medicine is an art as well as a science and nowhere is this demonstrated more clearly than in general practice. GPs are generalists, rather than specialists, which means they must embrace the whole of medicine instead of knowing about one clinical area in depth. In 2005 there were 42,876 GPs in the UK and 260 million doctor–patient consultations per annum (RCGP 2006).

The bulk of a GP's work is with patients with minor illnesses and chronic conditions, but they must retain their skills to deal with acute problems and medical emergencies as well. GPs have to make a quick and safe assessment of who is 'ill' and who 'not ill', who needs urgent admission to hospital and who can be reviewed at a later date. GPs are generally a patient's first point of contact with the NHS and so they come to see the doctor with undifferentiated and often confusing symptoms. It is part of the 'art' of practising medicine that helps the GP make sense of these symptoms and treat the patient appropriately. It requires a mix of excellent clinical knowledge, intuition and common sense to work out why the patient is there, what might be wrong and how to help. This is often different to the diagnostic process in the hospital setting because the GP may know the patient well and therefore understand their anxieties and beliefs, as well as their background and history. One of the pleasures of general practice is the continuity of care that can be offered to patients and the provision of ongoing support for them and their families over many years.

Roles of the GP

GPs have a role in the community as 'gatekeepers' to secondary and tertiary care in the UK. Only a small proportion of the patients who consult their GP (less than 15%) will be referred on to hospital or specialist services, but it is the GP who makes this decision with the patient and the rest of the team. Care for chronic conditions such as diabetes and asthma is now being managed by GPs and nursing staff in the practices in line with the govern-ment's plan to have a 'primary care led NHS'. According to the Royal College of General Practitioners (RCGP) figures in 2006, around 80% of GP consultations related to care of chronic disease.

In recent years, there has been a massive shift of resources from secondary to primary care and the new contract in 2004 (see below), gave GPs the choice and financial incentive to provide certain services at their practices (Directed Enhanced Services), above and beyond the basic patient care that all GPs must offer their patients.

Public health

We think of GPs mainly working on a one-to-one basis with the individual patient, but they also have a responsibility to the local population they serve. Their public health role includes the notification of certain diseases to the local public health laboratory and taking action if they are aware of clusters of disease or illness. An instance of this was when a GP in Cornwall recognized the symptoms of copper and lead poisoning in his patients (skin irritation, green hair and altered taste) and alerted the local authorities. This was the consequence of a major industrial accident in Camelford in July 1988, when toxic waste contaminated 20,000 peoples' water supplies.

Education

The word 'doctor' comes from the Latin *doctore* 'to teach'. GPs have always been involved in education, both of their patients and of other doctors training in general practice. A sea change in medical education, with much more emphasis on community-based training for students, has led to an increasing number of GPs teaching undergraduates, either on placement in their practices or in the medical school. A new respect has developed in academic medicine for general practice as a specialty in its own right, with its emphasis on a patient-centred approach and an holistic view of the patient. Postgraduate courses for GPs have been established to provide education and training for those interested in teaching on a regular basis.

Research

GPs have a long history of participating in and carrying out research, both in their own practices and in academic departments, which contributes to our understanding of the epidemiology of disease. Good examples of doctors who have been pioneers in this area are Professor Julian Tudor Hart who worked in Glyncorrwg West Glamorgan who proposed the concept of the 'inverse care law' in 1971, and the Scottish GP James McKenzie in the late 1890s. Linked to this tradition of research has been the development of health promotion and disease prevention in primary care. Every day in general practice GPs and nurses give advice to patients and carry out screening procedures (such as cervical smears, blood tests, child health surveillance and blood pressure checks), which contribute to improving the health of the nation as a whole, as well as the health of the patients concerned.

Advocacy

On an individual basis, GPs often act as patient advocates and point out local health inequalities, such as the problems that arise for asylum seekers accessing appropriate primary and secondary care, or the difficulties encountered by the elderly in isolated rural communities. GPs may liaise with hospital staff to speed up investigations or outpatient appointments on behalf of a patient, or write letters in support of rehousing. Many benefits from the government such as disability or carer's allowances require information from the patient's GP and filling in these applications makes up part of the daily work of a doctor in general practice. GPs can become involved in lobbying the government to change health policy to meet the needs that they perceive on a daily basis in the area where they work.

Government regulation

Until 2004, GPs were 'independent contractors' with the government, but there has been an increasing concern about the need to regulate general practice and this led to the introduction of a new GP contract. Through this, the government has attempted to standardize the care offered to patients across the UK. A large part of this contract lists certain 'targets' for patient care that should be met. These are arranged in four domains: clinical, organizational, additional and patient experience. The clinical targets listed in the Quality Outcomes Framework (QoF) include tasks such as monitoring blood pressure, carrying out medication reviews and performing regular specific blood tests and examinations relevant to

chronic conditions such as asthma and diabetes. Screening and immunization programmes also form part of the QoF targets, and practices that manage to monitor and/or screen a high percentage of their patients reap good financial rewards. Organizational targets include access issues and appointment waiting times.

The Directed Enhanced Services form part of the 'additional' domain of the contract and include the new 'choose and book' system, which gives the patient a choice of specialist and hospital, as well as an appointment time to suit them. (Of course, this is usually only available in well-resourced areas with several secondary and tertiary referral centres.) GPs can also opt into providing Local Enhanced Services which have been identified as necessary to meet local need by the Primary Care Organization (PCO). These might be minor surgery sessions, performing IUCD insertions or urea breath testing, for which there is an extra payment available to boost the practice income.

Information technology

Computerization has revolutionized primary care in many ways and is now virtually universal in GP practices. It helps to ensure that there is valid clinical and population data with appropriate contractual reimbursement and commissioning of services. The Read coding system, which most GPs use for classifying symptoms and diseases, also helps to ensure accurate recording of clinical information and aids communication within the primary health care team. In 2000, the government removed the legal requirement for paper-based notes. In 2010, it plans to introduce the NHS Spine, a national database of electronic care records for all patients in England and forming the core of the NHS Care Records Service (NHS CRS). The theory is that 'whenever and wherever a patient seeks care from the NHS in England, the staff treating them will have secure access to a summary of information to help with diagnosis and care' (NHS spine factsheet). The word 'secure' is crucial here as there are concerns about patient confidentiality and what would happen if the IT system failed or was tampered with in some way.

Decision support tools are being widely introduced in new software programs. These provide a way in which clinical outcomes in a particular condition can be predicted, based on an analysis of individual patient factors such as weight, family history and blood test results. They can lead to recommendations of treatment that are individually tailored, based on the latest evidence base. For example, the cardiovascular risk assessment tool shows the percentage risk of a patient experiencing a cardiovascular event in the next 5 years based on various parameters such as lipid profile, smoking history, age and sex.

However, there is a danger that such tools can replace common sense and clinical judgement and lead to 'automatism' on the part of the GP. Nothing can or should replace the therapeutic relationship between the doctor and patient which is maintained by clinical competence, good communication between both parties and mutual respect. Computers can be useful to share understanding with the patient and educate them about their condition, but they can also hinder sympathetic listening and explaining. A doctor who is more interested in tapping in information and gazing at a screen will soon lose the trust and respect of the individual in front of them.

In the General Medical Council's (GMC) *Duties of a Doctor*, it is stipulated that doctors must give information to patients in a way that they can understand, as well as involving them in decisions about their care, ensuring confidentiality and treating all patients with respect and dignity.

Monitoring quality

Repeat prescribing, patient records and practice statistics are usually all held on the practice computer system and this makes it much easier to keep accurate figures from year to year. The new GP contract requires that all practices carry out regular audits on the care they are offering to their patients and there are financial penalties for those who are not meeting the high standards set. Besides these patient and disease audits, analysis of prescribing patterns or the number of blood tests ordered can give practitioners useful information to discuss and change their practice to ensure a consistent and effective approach to patients. As practices grow and the complexity of the information they hold increases, so do the number of administrative staff needed to handle this information. Practice managers may have IT training, but in some of the larger primary care organizations, there may be one or two employees whose sole responsibility is to maintain and update the computerized records and carry out regular audits and research.

Evidence-based medicine

GPs now have access to a wealth of web-based resources on clinical practice, including local referral and management protocols, national guidelines and evidence-based systematic reviews. They keep up-to-date with the latest information on acute and chronic diseases by using web-based e-journals or websites that condense and summarize important clinical data (e.g. Prodigy, Bandolier, Cochrane collaboration websites). It is part of a GP's responsibility to be engaged in continuous personal and professional development so that they can offer the best quality care to their patients. The annual appraisal system for GPs provides one way in which doctors are monitored by their peers to ensure they are practising safe clinical medicine, can identify any gaps in their knowledge and are behaving professionally and with probity at all times (see GMC 2006).

The National Institute for Health and Clinical Excellence (NICE) produces regular guidelines on the treatment of conditions, based on the latest research evidence, which all GPs are expected to read and follow in their daily practice. There may also be local protocols or prescribing guidelines in some areas, which have been developed by a team of specialists and primary care health professionals to ensure consistency and quality of treatment.

Teamwork

The Primary Health Care Team is a broad term that refers to anyone working in or alongside a practice that is responsible to and for the patients. This commonly includes other health professionals such as nurses, midwives, health visitors and district nurses. It may also include people with specialist training such as the local pharmacist, social worker or a member of a community agency such as Age Concern. The point is that to offer holistic and individual care for a patient, the GP may be only one of many people involved, although he or she may have a leading role within the team as it is the GP who has overall responsibility for the patients on their list.

In the last 20 years, many practice nurses have undergone further training in the management of chronic disease and are taking over this role from doctors. In most practices, clinics in asthma, diabetes and cardiovascular disease are run by trained nursing staff, often working from locally agreed protocols, with reference to the GP only when there are problems or clinical decisions that the nurse is not able to make. Nurse practitioners are a relatively new role. They are often practice nurses who have received postgraduate training to diagnose and prescribe for certain conditions. In some practices, they may triage calls, hold surgeries and deal with many of the patients with minor illnesses and trauma who come to the surgery.

The larger the practice, the more likely it is that they will employ other professionals who can offer their services to the patient population. This might include physiotherapy, counselling, osteopathy or podiatry. There is a move to develop specialist services within primary care and some practices hold specialist monthly clinics at which one of the hospital consultants will see patients. Many GPs now have specialist training (General Practitioner with a Special Interest, GPwSI) and are able to offer services within their practice that were previously only available in hospital. An example of this might be a GPwSI who is trained in rheumatology and can diagnose and treat connective tissue diseases or give joint injections.

Environment

Practising as a GP in the inner city is very different to working in a remote rural setting and GPs need different skills depending on the environment in which they work. In the inner city, the GP may be dealing with a high turnover of patients and social issues such as housing, overcrowding and poverty may affect the health needs of the community they serve. However, there is likely to be a hospital nearby and ready access to laboratory and X-ray facilities, specialist services and advice from colleagues working in the area.

In contrast, a GP working in the Scottish Highlands may cover a large rural area with patients living in very isolated conditions. The GP must be able to deal with medical emergencies without the luxury of an ambulance round the corner or access to investigations at a local laboratory. This will make a difference to the sort of equipment and drugs he or she needs in their car or doctor's bag. Of course, poverty and deprivation exist in rural areas as well as in our cities, but the GP in such an area is likely to deal with a more stable population and one in which he or she has a central role and is known and recognized by everyone in the community.

It is one of the joys of general practice that a doctor can choose the environment they want to work in and the variety and interest will be completely different from another practice only a few miles away.

Changing face of primary care

Patients are better informed and have higher expectations of their doctors and the health service than ever before, which puts greater demands on GPs and their practices than in the past. Equally, GPs have changed their expectations about what hours of work they want to do and services they will provide. There are diminishing numbers of single-handed GPs and most doctors now work in partnerships with others, some in very large organizations that may serve a patient population of several thousand. Continuity of care is more difficult and while it remains an aspiration, both doctors and patients move around more than in the past. An increasing number of GPs hold salaried posts or are self-employed as non-principals. More doctors are choosing to work part-time (10% of GPs in 1995 and 25% in 2005 according to the RCGP 2006), and want to achieve a work–family–leisure balance that protects them against illness, alcohol and drug misuse and burnout.

Out-of-hours care

Historically, GPs have provided out-of-hours cover for their patients, usually on a rota basis between partners or between several local practices, who have shared the task of dealing with patients needing medical attention in the evenings or at weekends. The new contract in 2004 enabled GPs to opt out of doing any out-of-hours work and this responsibility was delegated to the primary care trusts. Inevitably, this has had an impact on continuity of care with few patients now seeing their own doctor outside of surgery opening hours.

In 1998, a 24-hour telephone health advice service (NHS Direct) provided mainly by nurses, was introduced by the government to increase patient access to advice and treatment for common conditions and to reduce the pressure on GP appointments. There is some evidence that the service is more costly and less efficient than spending the money on increasing the number of nurses within a practice who can triage patient calls and arrange urgent appointments if necessary (Richards *et al.* 2004). One study did show that there was a small decrease in the demand on out-of-hours general practice services after the introduction of NHS Direct (Munro *et al.* 2000).

NHS walk-in centres were also set up in 2000 to improve access to primary care services and take the pressure off GPs who were finding it difficult to meet the demand for doctor consultations. In January 2007 there were 66 of these centres in England (RCGP 2007). They are generally nurse-led, provide advice and treatment for minor illnesses and injuries and are open long hours. There has been much criticism that their establishment has led to an even more disparate health provision for patients with no continuity of care or satisfactory follow-up arrangements. Several studies have shown that walk-in centres have no impact on consultation rates at other health care providers (Hsu *et al.* 2003; Maheswaran *et al.* 2007).

Organization of primary health care

It is impossible to provide a comprehensive description of the organization of primary health care within the NHS as the pace of change is relentless. Many GPs are exhausted and frustrated by government demands to provide more services and documentation while they struggle to see patients and make informed clinical judgements. By the time this book is published, new structures and arrangements will have been developed. A recent change has been the emergence of private health care organizations that have taken on running some GP practices, seizing the opportunity to provide the Enhanced Services mentioned above. Many health professionals in primary care despair of the introduction of market forces into the NHS with companies 'bidding' to provide sexual health screening or phlebotomy services, for instance. There is a danger that if GPs do not provide such services or pay other GPs to do this in a particular locality, the primary care trust may commission the work from the private sector which could eventually render the GP bankrupt.

Primary care trusts

There has been a push by the government to move health services from the more expensive secondary and tertiary care centres into primary care, with GP practices under pressure to provide more and more services for their patients in the community. In 2002, 303 primary care trusts (PCTs) were set up to plan, provide and commission health services from health providers, based on the needs of the local population and with the aim of improving the health of that population. Their remit was also to integrate health and social services. To meet these aims, PCTs were allocated 75% of the NHS budget and overseen by the larger primary care organizations (PCOs). In the future, PCTs may disappear and be integrated into fewer regionally based PCOs.

While this major reorganization of general practice has led to an improvement of the services offered to patients in some parts of the country, several PCTs have overspent their budget and have had to cut back on the facilities they offer or cancel contracts with health providers. PCTs will now take over the health and social needs assessment process of the local population and commission services. For example, in a locality with many elderly patients, it might be appropriate for more of the PCT budget to be spent on podiatry and audiology services than on fertility or drug and alcohol services.

Practice-based commissioning

Practice-based commissioning is another model that the government plans to introduce shortly. This will mean that individual practices are allocated their own budget (global sum) to buy services directly from service providers, including the private sector, ostensibly to improve the quality and range of services available for their patients in addition to those already provided by the PCT. The government see this as a way to reduce the spiralling cost of the NHS. Making practices pay for services out of their own budget should motivate them to decrease the number of unnecessary tests or referrals and so cut costs. It is highly debatable whether this will encourage the practice of good medicine if the GP is constantly working out the price of investigations and treatment for a patient and could easily interfere with acting in the patient's 'best interests'.

Doctor–patient relationship

At the centre of general practice has always been the therapeutic doctor–patient relationship. From the point of view of the GP, it is a unique privilege getting to know patients over time, accompanying them on their journey through health and sickness and trying to ensure the best outcomes for that individual's mental and physical health. Anyone with a curiosity about people, a wish to experience clinical variety and the daily challenge of making sense of undifferentiated symptoms will find general practice one of the most interesting and unpredictable specialties in medicine.

References

General Medical Council (GMC). (2006) *Duties of a doctor.* www.gmc-uk.org/guidance/good_medical_practice/duties_of_a_doctor.asp Accessed on 28 August 2007.

General Medical Council (GMC). (2006) *Good medical practice.* www.gmc-uk.org/guidance/good_medical_practice/index.asp Accessed on 19 February 2008.

Hsu, R.T., Lambert, P.C., Dixon-Woods, M. & Kurinczuk, J.L. (2003) Effect of NHS walk-in centre on local primary healthcare services: before and after observational study. *BMJ* **326**, 530.

Maheswaran, R., Pearson, T., Munro, J., Jiwa, M., Campbell, M.J. & Nicholl, J. (2007) Impact of NHS walk-in centres on primary care access times: ecological study. *BMJ* **334**, 838.

Munro, J., Nicholl, J., O'Cathain, A. & Knowles, E. (2000) Impact of NHS Direct on demand for immediate care: observational study. *BMJ* **321**, 150–153.

NHS spine factsheet. www.connectingforhealth.nhs.uk/resources/comms_tkjune05/spine_factsheet.pdf Accessed on 26 August 2007.

National Institute for Health and Clinical Excellence (NICE) guidelines. www.nice.org.uk Accessed on 21 August 2007.

Richards, D.A., Godfrey, L., Tawfik, J., Ryan, M., Meakins, J., Duttob, E., *et al.* (2004) NHS Direct versus general practice based triage for same day appointments in primary care: cluster randomised controlled trial. *BMJ* **329**, 774.

Royal College of General Practitioners (RCGP). (2006) *Key Demographic Statistics from UK General Practice.* www.rcgp.org.uk/pdf/ISS_info_01_Jul06.pdf Accessed on 26 August 2007.

Royal College of General Practitioners (RCGP). (2007) *The Primary Care Practice and its Team.* www.rcgp.org.uk/pdf/ISS_info_21_Feb07.pdf Accessed on 20 February 2008.

Approach to the patient

Initial impression

In general practice first impressions are very important. A GP may see 20 or more patients in a surgery and appointments are rarely more than 10 minutes long. It is a very short time in which to gather information, examine and treat the individual in front of you. One of the skills that a GP develops is close observation of the patient from the moment they enter the room:

• How do they look?
• What are they wearing and are they unkempt?
• How are they walking?
• Are they nursing an injured limb or hiding a skin rash?
• Do they seem anxious or depressed?
• Are they ill or in pain?

A huge amount of information can be gathered by simply watching and taking note of how the patient appears in the seconds it takes them to walk through the door and sit down in the chair.

The patient-centred approach

The 'patient-centred approach' is the model used in medical education and GP training that describes what many GPs have done routinely for years. The emphasis is on listening attentively, not interrupting the patient and trying to understand the impact of any symptoms on that individual's life. It also involves finding out what the patient is concerned about, their understanding of what is wrong with them and their beliefs about how the problem occurred and what might be done to help. It is only after all this information has been gathered that the doctor negotiates a plan with the patient about investigation, treatment and follow-up.

As the RCGP's *A career in general practice* (2007) states: 'GPs are personal doctors, primarily responsible for the provision of comprehensive and continuing medical care to patients, irrespective of age, sex or illness. In negotiating medical plans with patients, they take account of physical, psychological, social/cultural factors, using the knowledge and trust engendered by a familiarity with past care, and an extensive understanding of medical conditions.'

The doctor-centred approach

The 'doctor-centred' approach is in contrast with the above and is seen as potentially damaging to the therapeutic relationship because it ignores the important psychosocial aspects of illness and disease and concentrates on a narrower biomedical view of the world. However, patients come to see doctors because of their clinical expertise and knowledge and want informed decisions to be made about their diagnosis and treatment. Doctors should not shy away from making these decisions, but in a patient-centred approach these are openly discussed and explained to reach 'shared understanding' with the patient, as opposed to the doctor dictating treatment and behaviour to them.

The GP is also an 'educator' and a great deal of time is spent with patients giving advice, answering queries, explaining medicines, diseases and procedures, reassuring patients and their families and providing support during distressing episodes of mental and physical illness. This role is a routine aspect of providing good clinical care and ensuring a holistic approach.

Safety and confidentiality

Patient safety is paramount and includes not just the clinical decisions that a GP might make about the patient, but also the wider working environment, communication issues, emergency drug storage and computer maintenance. Safety has become even more important as services have shifted from hospitals to the community and care for patients is delivered by a network of teams, individuals and practices. Research into patient safety has shown wide variation in error rates across the UK, the most common error being a failure or delay in diagnosis. In 2001, the National Patient Safety Agency (NPSA) was launched. It identified seven key areas of activity for primary care in 2005:

Confidentiality is another crucial principle that governs GP–patient consultations. GPs are privy to all sorts of information and may treat several members of the same family. The GMC's *Duties of a doctor* states that doctors must respect patients' right to confidentiality (except when there is serious risk to the patient or others) and never discriminate unfairly against patients or colleagues. It can be difficult for GPs always to adhere to these duties as they will undoubtedly come across patients (and colleagues) whose behaviour or attitude they disapprove of, or individuals they do not like. It is part of acting in a 'professional' manner to put aside any negative emotional responses and try to treat all patients with the same courtesy, consideration and clinical expertise.

Dealing with uncertainty

General practice is often the first port of call for patients and they may come with an array of symptoms and signs that do not fit easily into one disease entity. The GP must be able to deal with a degree of uncertainty about what is wrong with the patient and be aware that social and psychological factors may be as important as the physical problem. A watchful 'wait and see' approach with follow-up in a few days can be very helpful, unless of course the patient is obviously ill.

Home visits constitute another challenge in terms of diagnosis and treatment and the 'doctor's bag' should be equipped with all the necessary tools and drugs for investigation and treatment in the patient's home (see Appendix for list of contents).

History and examination

As with all medical specialties, the routine approach to the patient in general practice involves finding out the patient's reason for attendance, their symptoms and concerns and performing a physical examination to confirm or exclude different diagnoses.

Time constraints in the GP consultation mean that a full systems review and examination is not appropriate or necessary and GPs tend to do 'focused' histories and only examine the part of the patient that is relevant.

When medical students first spend time in primary care, they may be surprised and critical of the GP and think they are not being thorough enough in their history-taking or examination of the patient. It takes time to appreciate the considerable skill of the GP who can hone in on the problem and make informed clinical judgements about what is wrong with the patient, often based on extensive experience and knowledge about the individual in front of them.

Examinations in general practice must be carried out preserving the patient's dignity at all times and offering a chaperone if appropriate. Patients from different cultural backgrounds will have different expectations about what is acceptable in terms of undressing and allowing the doctor to examine certain parts of the body. The gender of the doctor may be crucial and ideally all practices should be able to offer their patients a choice of male or female GP to consult. Doctors of both sexes are legally required to offer a chaperone for many physical examinations. They should record in the notes that this has been done and if the patient has chosen to decline the offer for a third party to be present.

Preventive medicine

General practice often involves diagnosis and treatment but much of the everyday work is to do with primary and secondary prevention. A great deal of screening of patients is carried out for conditions such as high blood pressure, diabetes or cancer with appropriate advice, treatment or referral if these diseases are found. Secondary prevention, often involving medication and regular blood test monitoring, is routine for patients with chronic diseases with the aim of avoiding or delaying the complications that can ensue. Most screening is opportunistic, but some national programmes exist such as cervical screening for all women aged 25–65 years, most of which is carried out in primary care settings. The GP has an important role in many preventive measures such as advice on safe drinking limits, encouraging smoking cessation and screening for mental health problems to identifying those at risk of suicide so that urgent referral and intervention can be arranged.

Investigations and treatment

The local environment of the practice will dictate what investigations can be done within the surgery, ordered at a nearby hospital or clinic or require the patient to travel many miles for specialist tests. Blood tests, swabs, urine and faecal samples are usually easily dealt with by the practice, which will send them off to the nearest laboratory and receive the results electronically or through the post. A diminishing number of GPs will have a microscope and the training to look at microbiology swabs or urine samples to diagnose common infections such as vaginal candidiasis or *Escherichia coli* urinary infections. Urinanalysis dipsticks are an everyday diagnostic tool and glucometers provide a quick way to check a patient's blood sugar level. Many practices have ECG machines and defibrillators, ultrasound Doppler devices as well as portable nebulizers for treating acute asthmatic attacks.

The surgery will have an emergency bag with drugs and equipment for treating a range of life-threatening conditions which will include airways of different sizes, intravenous cannulae and fluids and medicines for treating conditions such as acute anaphylaxis, post-partum haemorrhage, myocardial infarction, meningitis, injuries and hypoglycaemia (see Appendix on p. 183 for full list).

Most GPs do not have direct access to magnetic resonance imaging (MRI) or computed tomography (CT) scans, colonoscopies or more invasive investigations such as angiography or arthroscopy. At the moment, a patient who requires any of these must be referred to secondary care or a management centre which decides from the patient's history and findings how urgent the investigation is and puts the patient on a waiting list accordingly.

Services in primary care are expanding and increasing numbers of GPs are training as specialists in certain fields. Practices are purchasing more sophisticated diagnostic equipment such as X-ray facilities, ultrasound and endoscopes and often employ other health professionals who can offer physiotherapy, counselling or complementary therapies such as acupuncture or homeopathy. These extra services may attract income under the Local Enhanced Services if they have been identified as serving the local population need by the primary care trust.

Dangers of under and over investigation

In considering the patient in front of them, the GP must decide the probability of serious disease and how far to investigate the problem with further tests. It is negligent to ignore or underrate a patient's symptoms or signs, but the converse is also true and over investigation can lead to making the patient unnecessarily anxious, as well as wasting NHS resources. In all cases, the GP must use his or her clinical judgement, based on their knowledge and experience, to decide what is appropriate and safe for the individual patient.

Teamwork

While GPs are legally and morally responsible for looking after their patients, they rely heavily on nursing colleagues to share this responsibility and on administrative staff for the day-to-day running of the practice. To offer the best care to patients, teamwork and good communication between the health professionals involved is essential. Some practices will have health visitors, district nurses and midwives attached to them, whereas other practices may rely on a local nursing team based elsewhere, who work with several GPs in the area. Whatever arrangement exists, patient care is delivered by several different health workers, particularly in the case of elderly patients with multiple medical and social problems. Regular meetings within the practice to plan and coordinate the care delivered are an important aspect of patient safety and satisfaction.

References

General Medical Council (GMC). (2006) *Duties of a doctor.* www.gmc-uk.org/guidance/good_medical_practice/duties_of_a_doctor.asp Accessed on 28 August 2007.

Royal College of General Practitioners (RCGP). (2007) *A career in general practice: education, training and professional development in the UK.* www.rcgp.org.uk/pdf/ISS_info_Careers07.pdf Accessed on 28 August 2007.

National Patient Safety Agency (NPSA). *Seven steps to patient safety in primary care.* www.npsa.nhs.uk/health/resources/7steps?contented=2664 Accessed on 28 September 2007.

Clinical overview

GPs see only a small proportion of health problems experienced by the population at large and the majority of symptoms are managed by self-care. This includes self-medication, advice from family, friends or the local pharmacist and using alternative or complementary therapies. Symptoms are common, but only a small number of these result in a consultation with a doctor. So the question then arises: when and why do people choose to see their GP? The reasons are manifold and complex, including perception of the severity of the symptoms, their duration and how much they interfere with everyday life. Consultation rates are highest for the under-5s and the over-75s, reflecting the higher morbidity and mortality rates in these ages (Morbidity Statistics from General Practice 1991–1992).

Environment

Social deprivation is still a major cause of morbidity and mortality, with circulatory and smoking-related diseases forming the most common reason for death or disability. There are many reasons for this but income, in particular, is closely related to health. In the UK, the gap between rich and poor has widened, with more people living on less than 50% of the average income than 20 years ago (Simon *et al.* 2005). Unemployment is another important predictor of illness and disease. It has long been recognized as a risk factor for poor health, with increased rates of depression and ischaemic heart disease as well as mortality from coronary vascular disease, cancer, suicide, accidents and violence. The medical conditions that GPs see in their surgery depend very much on the demographics of the environment they are working in, the local socioeconomic situation and rates of employment.

Statistics

Over 95% of the British population are registered with a GP and in 2005 there were 42,876 registered GPs. There has been a steady rise in the number of GPs per 100,000 people in England but this figure does not take into account the fact that there has been a growth in the number of GPs who are now part-time in general practice (RCGP 2006). GPs carry out nearly 300 million consultations per annum, of which over 80% take place at the surgery, 10% are on the telephone and around 3% are at other locations (The Information Centre 2007). GP home visits have decreased substantially from 22% of all consultations in 1971 to 5% in 2002–2003 (Office for National Statistics 2004).

The average number of GP consultations per person has remained at about four per year since 1972, but the number of patients consulting the practice nurse has increased substantially because of their role in health promotion and managing chronic disease (Table 1).

The detailed analysis of these figures in terms of age, gender and disease makes for fascinating reading, as well as the different consulting rates for the north and south of England, but there is not space to include the information here.

It is interesting that top of this list is the 'Supplementary classification of factors influencing health status and contact with health services' which covers reasons for attending the practice other than illness. Almost one-third of consultations fall into this category and reflect the vast amount of screening procedures, health promotion and preventive medicine that is carried out in primary care. Another point mentioned earlier in this introduction is that GPs see a great deal of undifferentiated 'illness' that cannot be classified into a 'disease' or well-recognized medical condition. This is reflected in the figure of 15% for the classification 'Symptoms, signs and ill-defined conditions'.

Of course, this data only provides a snapshot of 1% of the population seeing their GPs in England and Wales over the year that the information was collected (1991–1992). Each classification is not mutually exclusive and many patients consult with their doctor about several different problems at the same time. If a similar study was conducted now, consultations for certain conditions such

Table 1 Most common reasons for patients to consult their doctor. [From Morbidity Statistics from General Practice 1991–1992.]

	Percentage
Supplementary classification (immunization, health surveillance, antenatal and contraceptive care)	33
Respiratory problems (coughs and colds, asthma, bronchitis, chronic obstructive airways disease, emphysema)	31
Disorders of the nervous system (headache, ear and eye infections, migraine, dizziness)	17
Musculoskeletal problems (osteoarthritis, backache, joint pain, rheumatoid arthritis)	15
Skin disorders (eczema, psoriasis, acne)	15
Symptoms, signs and ill-defined conditions (dizziness, cough, rash, headache, dyspnoea, chest pain, nausea and vomiting, abdominal pain)	15
Injury and poisoning (fractures, sprains, strains, open wounds, contusions)	14
Infectious or parasitic diseases (*Candida*, herpes, dermatomycosis, warts, scabies, gastroenteritis)	14
Diseases of the genitourinary system (cystitis, pyelonephritis, pelvic inflammatory disease, prostatism, menopause)	11
Diseases of the digestive system (dyspepsia, oesophagitis, gastritis, gastric and duodenal ulcers, liver and gall bladder disease)	9
Disease of the circulatory system (hypertension, ischaemic heart disease, angina, cerebrovascular disease, myocardial infarction)	9
Mental illness (depression, anxiety, chronic fatigue, insomnia)	7
Endocrine, nutritional and metabolic diseases (diabetes, obesity, thyroid disease, gout)	4

as obesity and diabetes would have increased as these have become more prevalent and a major cause of morbidity in the last 15 years.

Women had a higher consultation rate than men for reasons classified as minor or intermediate and this is likely to still be the case. Many contacts are for contraception and antenatal care and not for illness as such. According to the 1991–1992 Morbidity Study, in all age groups, rates of illness classified as serious were similar for men and women.

Consultation rates were highest for children under 5 years, particularly for respiratory problems, ear infections and skin diseases. Among the elderly, many consulted the GP about circulatory disorders, respiratory and musculoskeletal problems, but they also attended frequently for preventive procedures such as immunizations and health checks.

Reasons for seeing the doctor
From the patient's point of view, Table 2 lists symptoms that were worrying enough to warrant a GP visit. Perhaps surprisingly, the lists are remarkably similar, showing that

Table 2 Ten most common presenting symptoms in the GP surgery. [From Morrell 1972.]

Males	Females
Cough	Cough
Rash	Rash
Sore throat	Sore throat
Abdominal pain	Spots, sores, ulcers
Bowel symptoms	Abdominal pain
Chest pain	Bowel symptoms
Back pain	Back pain
Spots, sores, ulcers	Chest pain
Headache	Gastric symptoms
Joint pain	Headache

both sexes worry about the same sort of symptoms, although a more detailed analysis is required to interpret these and explore the psychosocial aspects of each presentation.

A more recent, prospective 5-year cohort study of 738 patients from a suburban Manchester general practice (Kapur *et al.* 2005) found a higher consultation rate among women (as noted before) and gender differences in the reasons for consultation with the GP. Factors relating to psychological distress were more important for women whereas physical symptoms and cognitive factors were more important for men.

Evidence-based resources

GPs have access to a huge number of excellent evidence-based resources to aid them make well-informed clinical decisions with their patients, using the most up-to-date evidence.

Evidence-based medicine (EBM) involves the following approach:
• Identifying a clinical problem or need and turning it into an answerable question (e.g. what is the best first line treatment for simple urinary tract infection?)
• Finding the best evidence to answer this question
• Critically appraising the evidence for its usefulness and validity
• Applying the results in clinical practice
• Considering the outcomes and evaluating the results
This might mean an audit of all identified and treated urinary tract infections with a particular antibiotic over a specified period.

There is such a wealth of evidence available, how do GPs know which sources are reliable and valid? To help with this, there is a classification system for grading reliability of evidence (Table 3)

Critical appraisal is another tool in helping GPs interpret evidence in a systematic way and decide on its relevance, validity and whether the results are clinically useful for their patients. Appraisal tools can be downloaded from the Critical Appraisal Skills Programme (CASP) developed by Oxford University which involves a step-based approach to reading material and analysing its reliability and validity. It can be accessed via the National Library for Health.

There are many internationally recognized sources of web-based information which can inform clinical practice such as the National Library for Health. The mission of the National Library for Health (NLH) is 'to help patients and professionals use best current knowledge in decision-making'. It includes a number of different resources including evidence-based reviews such as the Cochrane Library; the National Library of Guidelines; NICE; books and journals; and patient resources.

Commonly used and respected electronic sources are listed in Box 1 and include websites with clinical guidelines. Some of these are also contained within the NLH.

Electronic bibliographical databases are also useful tools for finding the evidence behind clinical questions. Medline and Embase are two examples of these. Medline covers the whole field of medicine and Embase provides information on drugs and pharmacology. These and others can be found through NLH.

Bandolier and Prodigy both pride themselves on producing succinct, easy to read and understand clinical evidence that is of practical use to the busy GP. There are many barriers to why GPs do not always use EBM and these are summarized in an article from a study carried out in Australia (Belsey & Snell 2001). These included lack of Internet access, low understanding of EBM terms,

Table 3 Classification system for grading reliability of evidence. [After Belsey & Snell 2001.]

Grade A	Ia Meta-analysis of randomized controlled trials
	Ib Strong evidence from at least one randomized controlled trial of a reasonable size
Grade B	IIa Evidence from well-designed non-randomized trials (e.g. case-controlled or cohort study)
	IIb Evidence from well-designed quasi-experimental study
	III Evidence from well-designed non-experimental descriptive study from more than one study or research group (e.g. comparative studies, case studies, correlation studies)
Grade C	IV Opinions of respected authorities based on clinical evidence and descriptive studies or reports of expert committees

---

Box 1 Commonly used electronic sources of clinical information

http://www.jr2.ox.ac.uk/bandolier	Bandolier: Evidence-based thinking about health care
http://www.besttreatments.net/btgeneric/home/jsp	BMJ best treatments
http://www.clinicalevidence.bmj.com	Clinical Evidence (BMJ Publishing)
http://www.cochranelibrary.com	Cochrane library
http://www.ebm.bmj.com	Evidence-based medicine
http://www.gpnotebook.co.uk	GP encyclopaedia on-line
http://www.library.nhs.uk	National Electronic Library for Health
http://www.nice.nhs.uk	National Institute for Health and Clinical Excellence
http://www.npc.co.uk/merec_index.htm	National Prescribing Centre – MeReC Bulletin
http://www.york.ac.uk/inst/crd	NHS Centre for Reviews and Dissemination
http://www.nzgg.org.nz	New Zealand Guidelines Group
http://www.cks.library.nhs.uk	Prodigy: Clinical Knowledge Summaries
http://www.ncbi.nlm.nih.gov	PubMed: A service of the US National Library of Medicine
http://www.sign.ac.uk	Scottish Intercollegiate Guidelines Network

---

time, money and skills. However, the new generation of doctors are being trained to use EBM resources as a matter of course and critically appraise new information in a systematic and logical fashion. There are those who argue against slavish devotion to EBM as it can interfere with the doctor–patient relationship and intuitive clinical reasoning and judgement. A balance is needed between using EBM resources which give the generalist summarized recommendations about clinical problems and applying them to the individual patient in front of them, with the patients' particular symptoms, psychosocial circumstances and idiosyncratic reactions to medications. This is the 'art' of practising medicine and one of its most rewarding aspects in general practice.

References

Belsey, J. & Snell, T. (2001) *What is evidence-based medicine?* www.jr2.ox.ac.uk/bandolier/band92/692–6.html Accessed on 2 October 2007.

Critical Appraisal Skills Programme (CASP). http://www.phru.nhs.uk/casp Accessed on 4 October 2007.

Kapur, N., Hunt, I., Lunt, M., McBeth, J., Creed, F. & Macfarlane, G. (2005) Primary care consultation predictors in men and women: a cohort study. *British Journal of General Practice* **55**, 108–113.

Royal College of General Practitioners (RCGP). (2006) *Key Demographic Statistics from UK General Practice.* www.rcgp.org.uk/pdf/ISS_fact_06.KeyStats.pdf Accessed on 4 October 2007.

Office for National Statistics. (July 2004) *General Household Survey for GP Consultation Data.* www.statistics.gov.uk.

Morbidity Statistics from General Practice, 4th National Study 1991–1992. Office of Population Censuses and Surveys Series MB3 no 5. www.statistics.gov.uk/downloads/theme_health/MB5No3.pdf Accessed on 2 October 2007.

Morrell, D.C. (1972) Symptom interpretation in general practice. *Journal of the Royal College of Practitioners* **22**, 297.

Simon, C., Everitt, H. & Kendrick, T. (2005) *Oxford Handbook of General Practice.* Oxford University Press, Oxford.

The Information Centre. (2007) *Trends in Consultation Rates in General Practice 1995–2006.* www.ic.nhs.uk/statistics-and-data-collections/primary-care/general-practice/trends-in-consultation-rates-in-general-practice 1995–2006 Accessed on 2 December 2007.

Case 1 A 40-year-old female smoker with a chest infection

Mrs Audrey Cartwright, 40, is a sheltered housing warden, and comes to see you with a cough which she has had for 2 weeks. You know she is a smoker, of 20/day for 20 years. There is no record of recent smoking cessation advice being given. It appears that she came in last winter with a cough.

What other questions do you want to ask?
- Duration of the cough?
- Is the cough productive, if so of what?
- Any reduced exercise tolerance?
- Any shortness of breath?
- Has she experienced chest pain, on coughing or inspiration?
- Any symptoms?

She confirms that she has had the cough for 2 weeks, it is productive in nature, of green and yellow foul-tasting sputum. She does not feel able run up the stairs as well as she did. She says she begins coughing and then becomes short of breath. She occasionally feels pain on coughing and this is sharp in nature. It is in her back and this is not associated with breathing in. She has not noticed any blood in her sputum. She feels tired because the cough does tend to wake her during the night. She had no symptoms until 2 weeks previously and thinks of herself as generally fit and healthy.

What is your differential diagnosis?
- Lower respiratory tract infection (LRTI) – viral
- LRTI – bacterial
- Pneumonia
- Underlying lung disease

How would you proceed?
She consents for an examination, and she was apyrexial, pulse 88 beats/min, no evidence of respiratory distress, respiratory rate of 14 breaths/min, no evidence of tonsillitis and her chest was clear on auscultation with good air entry throughout and no wheeze.

She tells you that she expects antibiotics as they are the only thing that shifts it and she is unable to take time of work as there is no cover for her.

What are your reasons for each diagnosis and the possible treatment strategies?
Viral LRTI
The supporting features are the short duration of illness, without evidence of underlying lung disease and an essentially normal examination.

The treatment options include symptomatic treatment or delayed prescription for antibiotics (a prescription to be used at a later date if symptoms persist).

Bacterial LRTI
Supporting this diagnosis are the discoloured foul-tasting sputum, reduced exercise tolerance and the possibility of underlying lung disease as a long-term smoker.

Treatment options include delayed prescription for antibiotics, antibiotics and symptomatic treatment.

Community acquired pneumonia
This is unlikely because of the absence of systemic illness and the absence of chest signs.

What are the other considerations in this situation?
- Patient preference and expectation
- Overuse of antibiotics in general practice
- Emergence of antibiotic resistance

You are aware of her expectations and priorities and decide to offer her a delayed prescription of an antibiotic.

Which antibiotic do you choose and for how long do you give it?
The considerations are:
- Likely pathogens
- Patterns of resistance in your area

- Drug allergies
- Weight of the patient
- Possible renal or hepatic impairment
- Other medications, including over-the-counter remedies

If you are considering a bacterial cause, the two most common pathogens are *Streptococcus pneumoniae* and *Haemophilus influenzae*. Unless there is local resistance to either microbe, amoxicillin and doxycycline are drugs of choice (Jones *et al.* 2004, section 2.2). The usual dosage of amoxicillin is 500 mg t.i.d. for 5 days. The usual dosage of doxycycline is 200 mg on day 1, then 100 mg once daily for 6 days.

How do you negotiate a delayed (back pocket) prescription?

By using a delayed prescription you aim to reduce the number of antibiotics used in acute LRTI, reduce antibiotic resistance, and reduce the need for medical intervention in subsequent episodes (Arroll 2003). There has been a systematic review of the use of delayed prescriptions and there was an overall reduction in the numbers of antibiotics used, and there was a delay in prescription use of 1–7 days (Arroll *et al.* 2003).

You initially start the discussion by summarizing both viewpoints. You understand her position, which is every year her chest infection clears up only with the use of antibiotics and she cannot afford time off work. Your position is that the chest infection is mild and will clear up of its own accord. You know antibiotics in this case will not shorten the duration of the illness, nor improve her symptoms any quicker (Jones *et al.* 2004, section 2.2).

You offer a prescription, to be filled on the basis of review in up to 3 days if symptoms persist or worsen. There must be a proviso that the patient should monitor and request review by a doctor if they become systemically unwell, have haemoptysis or have any other cause for concern. The patient may take the antibiotics rather than re-present for review.

Not all doctors advocate the use of delayed prescriptions, often because of the perception that they will be perceived in a negative light or that there is a higher associated medicolegal risk (Arroll 2003).

Is there an opportunity for health promotion?

This is a prime time for smoking cessation advice in the face of a condition where smoking is a contributory factor.

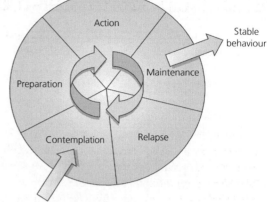

Figure 1 The cycle of change. Adapted from Prochaska and DiClemente (1984).

Assessing Mrs Cartwright's motivations for continuing smoking and barriers to change allow assessment of her within the 'cycle of change' (Fig. 1).

> She tells you she would like to stop and does recognize the health risks. She feels unable to at the moment as her husband also smokes, it is part of her rounds as the warden and she finds it a sociable pastime. She feels she is under too much pressure at work to consider it.

She is in the 'contemplation' stage of the cycle of change. You give her a leaflet from NHS Direct (Patient Information Leaflet – Quitting Smoking) stating the benefits of stopping and how to access NHS Smoking Cessation clinics.

> Outcome. Mrs Cartwright filled her prescription 2 days after the consultation. She continues to smoke.

References

Akkerman, A.E., Kuyvenhoven, M.M., van der Wouden, J.C. & Verheij, T.J.M. (2005) Prescribing antibiotics for respiratory tract infections by GPs: management and prescriber characteristics. *British Journal of General Practice* **55**, 114–118.

Arroll, B. (2003) Delayed prescriptions: can reduce antibiotic use in acute respiratory infections. *BMJ* **327**, 1361–1362.

Arroll, B., Kenealy, T. & Kerse, N. (2003) Do delayed prescriptions reduce antibiotic use in respiratory tract

PART 2: CASES

CASE REVIEW

LRTI is a cough accompanied by at least one of increased sputum production, dyspnoea, wheeze, chest pain or discomfort, in which the symptoms have been present for under 21 days and there is no obvious alternative explanation for the symptoms (e.g. sinusitis, asthma, cardiac disease; Holmes *et al.* 2001).

LRTI are the most common reason for presentation to the GP (up to 20% of all consultations; Akkerman *et al.* 2005), with this rate increasing over the past 10 years (McFarlane *et al.* 1997a), and up to 75% of these consultations result in an antibiotic prescription (McFarlane *et al.* 1997a). Up to half of these prescriptions are thought to be unnecessary (Akkerman *et al.* 2005).

There are many reasons for a prescription of an antibiotic to be generated, including patient pressure (Coenen *et al.* 2006), length of time the GP has been in practice (Akkerman *et al.* 2005), GP's perceived knowledge of respiratory tract infections (Akkerman *et al.* 2005), GP's perceived amount of time they have with each patient (Akkerman *et al.* 2005) and re-presentation within the same illness (Holmes *et al.* 2001; McFarlane *et al.* 1997a). Anecdotally, one may think that antibiotics are more likely to be prescribed on a Friday afternoon; however, this has not been supported (McFarlane *et al.* 1997b).

Information regarding the natural history of LRTI, and in particular the duration of the cough, may reduce the numbers of re-presentations within the same illness, thus reducing the number of second line antibiotics prescribed.

KEY POINTS

- Careful history and examination to establish a clear clinical picture
- Discussion regarding the reason for presentation now
- Incorporation of the patient's expectations into the management plan
- In this case, her expectations were based upon her social and occupational situation
- Overuse of antibiotics in general practice may be a result of overdiagnosis of bacterial LRTI, patient expectation, comorbid conditions (e.g. asthma and chronic obstructive pulmonary disease [COPD])

- There is increasing antibiotic resistance in the community
- There is high re-presentation rate within the same illness for cough
- Explanation of the natural history of the illness may reduce re-presentation
- Patient information leaflets may be useful is changing help-seeking behaviour
- Delayed prescription and follow-up may reduce the amount of antibiotics used

infections? A systematic review. *British Journal of General Practice* **53**, 871–877.

Coenen, S., Michiels, B., Renard, D., Denekens, J. & Van Royen, P. (2006) Antibiotic prescribing for acute cough: the effect of perceived demand. *British Journal of General Practice* **56**, 183–190.

Holmes, W.F., McFarlane, J.T., MacFarlane, R.M. & Hubbard, R. (2001) Symptoms, signs, and prescribing for acute lower respiratory tract illness. *British Journal of General Practice* **51**, 177–181.

Jones, R., Britten, N., Culpepper, L., Gass, D., Grol, R., Mant, D., *et al.* (eds.) (2004) *Oxford Textbook of Primary Medical Care*. Oxford University Press, Oxford.

McFarlane, J.T., Holmes, W.F. & MacFarlane, R.M. (1997a) Reducing reconsultations for acute lower respiratory tract illness with an information leaflet: a randomised controlled study of patients in primary care. *British Journal of General Practice* **47**, 719–722.

McFarlane, J.T., Lewis, S., McFarlane, R. & Holmes, W. (1997b) Contemporary use of antibiotics in 1089 adults presenting with acute lower respiratory tract illness in general practice in the UK: implications for developing management guidelines. *Respiratory Medicine* **91**, 427–434.

NHS Direct Patient Information Leaflets. www.cks. library.nhs.uk/patient_information_leaflet/smoking_ quitting Accessed on 21 May 2007.

Prochaska, J.O. & DiClemente, C.C. (1984) *The Transtheoretical Approach: Crossing Traditional Boundaries of Therapy*. Don Jones-Irwin, Homewood, IL.

Case 2 A 9-year-old asthmatic child

You are the duty (on-call) doctor for the surgery and are informed by the receptionists that there is an emergency home visit request for a 9-year-old boy, Jake, who is short of breath. He is a known asthmatic. You are in the middle of morning surgery.

What is your immediate reaction?

You need to triage the call and decide whether to call for an ambulance, visit the child at home immediately, visit the child after morning surgery or ask whoever is looking after the child to bring him in.

What information do you need to decide which option is most appropriate?

• What is the clinical state of the child?
• What is the past medical history – does Jake have a past diagnosis of asthma and/or a history of previous similar episodes and/or admissions to hospital?
• Who is with the child and what are their fears and concerns?
• Are they at home and have they any transport?
• Have they any prescription medicines, in particular asthma inhalers?

To find out this information you need to look at the medical notes and speak to whoever is looking after Jake.

His mother is worried and says that he has been unwell for a couple of days with a runny nose and a temperature. He has asthma and it is normally well controlled with him rarely needing to use his inhaler. In contrast, he has needed his inhaler several times during the last couple of days to control his wheeziness and cough. This morning he has already needed his inhaler four times and on each occasion the effects did not last long. He is on the sofa wrapped in a blanket.

His medical notes state that he is prescribed a salbutamol metered dose inhaler. He has not had any admissions to hospital.

Do you have enough information? What further questions would you ask to help assess his clinical state?

• Is he awake or asleep? Is he rousable if asleep?
• Is he talking? If so, is he able to speak full sentences or just single words?
• Is his breathing noisy or quiet?
• What is his colour?
• How long has he been like this?

You find out that he is sitting on the sofa and is able to talk short sentences. He sounds wheezy and looks flushed. He has been like this most of the morning.

You decide that his condition is not immediately life-threatening but could deteriorate quickly and so instruct the mother that you will attend, leaving surgery immediately.

Should she do anything while she is waiting?

Give him more puffs of his salbutamol inhaler via the spacer (up to 10 puffs). She should dial 999 if he suddenly deteriorates before you arrive.

What do you need to do before you leave the surgery?

• Tell the receptionists that you are leaving and ask them to inform the patients who are waiting
• Get a printout of your patient's summarized medical records
• Take your mobile phone so that you can be contacted and so that you can contact others
• Make sure that you know where you are going

What should you take with you?

Along with the routine items that you would expect to see in a doctor's bag you should take, as a minimum, a bronchodilator (e.g. salbutamol metered dose inhaler) and a spacer device. Some GPs also have access to portable nebulizers but evidence has shown that metered dose inhalers with spacers are as effective as nebulizers in delivering β_2-agonists (Closa *et al.* 1998). A peak flow meter would also be useful as it will help you to assess the severity of the episode.

On arrival at the house what are the most important things to do?

You need to assess Jake rapidly while putting him and his mother at ease. Anxiety will only make his condition worse.

How would you assess him?

You should assess the severity of his symptoms and clinical signs (Table 4), but it should be remembered that the signs can correlate poorly with the degree of airway obstruction (BTS, SIGN 2005). Normal values for respiratory rate and pulse rate can be found in the Appendix.

- Pulse rate
- Respiratory rate and degree of breathlessness
- Use of accessory muscles of respiration
- Amount of wheezing
- Degree of agitation and conscious level

A measurement of less than 50% of predicted or best peak flow with poor response after initial bronchodilator

is predictive of a prolonged asthma attack. The national guidelines suggest that peak flow should be attempted in all children aged over 5 years and the best of three readings taken but in practice, particularly if the child is unwell, this is not practical (BTS, SIGN 2005).

He has an audible wheeze and cough. He is fully conscious and able to talk in short sentences. He is slightly anxious. His respiratory rate is 27 breaths/min, pulse rate is 116 beats/ min and he is not using any accessory muscles of respiration. His peak flow is 54% of predicted.

Why is it important to classify how severe this asthma attack is?

By classifying the severity you can then decide on the correct treatment using the *BNF for Children* (2007) (Box 2). It can also be used as a prognostic indicator.

This attack is of moderate severity and so after checking your BNF you give him a further 10 puffs of salbutamol via his spacer. He becomes less wheezy and breathless, his respiratory rate drops to 22 breaths/min and his pulse rate is 98 beats/min. After only a few minutes his symptoms return and Jake and his mother are becoming more upset.

Table 4 Clinical signs. [After *BNF for Children* 2007.]

	Mild	Moderate	Severe	Life-threatening
Under 2 years	Cough, wheeze, no distress No cyanosis Normal respiration rate Speaking normally	Oxygen saturation >92% Audible wheezing Using accessory muscles to breathe Still feeding	Oxygen saturation <92% Cyanosis Marked respiratory distress Too breathless to feed	
2–5 years	Cough, wheeze, no distress No cyanosis Normal respiration rate Speaking normally	Oxygen saturation >92% No clinical features of severe asthma	Oxygen saturation <92% Too breathless to talk or eat Heart rate >130 beats/min Respiratory rate >50 breaths/min Use of accessory muscles of breathing	Oxygen saturation <92% Silent chest Poor respiratory effort Agitation or altered consciousness Cyanosis
5–18 years	Cough, wheeze, no distress No cyanosis Normal respiration rate Speaking normally	Oxygen saturation >92% Peak flow >50% best or predicted No clinical features of severe asthma	Oxygen saturation <92% Peak flow <50% best or predicted Too breathless to talk Heart rate >120 beats/min Respiratory rate >30 breaths/min Use of accessory muscles of breathing	Oxygen saturation <92% Peak flow <33% best or predicted Silent chest Poor respiratory effort Altered consciousness or cyanosis

Box 2 Treatment

Only the age group appropriate for Jake is included here. (After *BNF for Children* 2007.)

Mild to moderate exacerbation

Salbutamol aerosol inhaler 100 µg/inhalation

Child 2–18 years
- 1 puff every 15–30 s through a spacer up to max 10 puffs. Repeat after 20–30 min if necessary
- Short course of prednisolone should also be prescribed
- If response is poor or if a relapse occurs within 3–4 h send child to hospital

Severe or life-threatening

Send immediately to hospital. While waiting for transfer give either salbutamol as above or nebulized solution.

Child 2–18 years
- 2.5 mg every 20–30 min if necessary, or terbutaline 5 mg every 20–30 min if necessary
- If response to β_2-agonist is poor (while awaiting transfer to hospital) ipratropium nebulized solution 125–250 µg every 20–30 min if necessary
- Oxygen should be administered if you have it
- Prednisolone tablets or hydrocortisone injection also form part of the treatment regime although it is likely that these would not be administered in the community prior to admission

What do you do next?

His symptoms have returned quickly, reinforcing the instability of his condition. His mother is also having difficulty coping and so you calmly inform Jake and his mother that it would be best if he goes to hospital for further assessment and treatment.

Jake's mother starts crying and says that she has no car to get there. You calm her down saying that it is the best place for him. You explain that you will arrange for an ambulance and ask if there is anyone that she could call for support. She calls Jake's father who says that he will meet them at the hospital.

Jake stays in hospital for 48 h. During this time the diagnosis is confirmed and he is stabilized with oral steroids and regular bronchodilator nebulizers. He is discharged with no change to his medications from those that he had on admission.

Why should you arrange for a follow-up appointment?

To ensure that the family:
- Are happy with his current condition
- Understand his treatment plan, including triggers and their avoidance (e.g. infection, allergy, airborne chemicals, passive smoking, exercise)
- Know what to do if another attack occurs and when to seek medical help

Outcome. Unfortunately, this episode heralds the start of a deterioration in his condition and he requires the addition of inhaled steroids within a couple of months because he requires bronchodilators on a daily basis. He has another admission to hospital with an acute attack within 6 months and the paediatricians decide to follow him up as an outpatient.

References and further reading

British National Formulary for Children. (2007) Royal Pharmaceutical Society of Great Britain. RPS Publishing and BMJ Publishing Group, London.

British Thoracic Society, Scottish Intercollegiate Guidelines Network (BTS, SIGN). (2005) *British Guideline on the Management of Asthma*, Revised edition. http://www.brit-thoracic.org.uk/Guidelinessince%201997_asthma_html Accessed on 13 March 2007.

Closa, R.M., Ceballos, J.M., Gomez-Papi, A., Sanchez-Galiana, A., Gutierrez, C. & Marti-Henneber, C. (1998) Efficacy of bronchodilators administered by nebulisers versus spacers in infants with acute wheezing. *Pediatric Pulmonology* **26**, 344–348.

CASE REVIEW

Asthma is a chronic inflammatory disease affecting the lower airways manifesting as reversible airway obstruction and mucosal inflammation resulting in bronchoconstriction. It has a prevalence of 10–23% in England, with the number of cases being diagnosed rising year on year (NICE 2002).

Asthma is a very serious condition with acute asthma causing approximately 1000 deaths in the UK per year (Currie *et al.* 2005). 'Regard each emergency consultation as being for acute severe asthma. Failure to respond adequately at any time requires immediate transfer to hospital.' (*BNF for Children* 2007, p. 165).

We know that diagnosis is not always simple but it should be suspected in any child with an audible wheeze, recurrent cough and breathlessness with acute exacerbations. The diagnosis can be confirmed in schoolchildren by peak flow variability or tests of bronchial hyper-reactivity (BTS, SIGN 2005).

Throughout this case different guidelines have been mentioned. National guidelines are developed by experts to help clinicians to diagnose and manage conditions using the best evidence available. Asthma guidelines are readily available in the *BNF* helping the clinician to assess the severity of the condition and to give the appropriate acute and long-term treatment.

In this case Jake's follow-up after discharge was mentioned. This is to ensure:

1 That the parents and child have a good understanding of the illness and the medication. Good education will result in improved symptom control, self-management and re-attendance rates (BTS, SIGN 2005). Education should include discussion of the avoidance of precipitants. These include infection, allergy, passive smoking and exercise (NICE 2002)
2 The correct type of inhaler is assessed so that the dose of drug entering the lungs is maximized (NICE 2002)
3 Action plans are written. They improve health outcomes and they should be focused on individual needs (BTS, SIGN 2005)

The National Service Framework flow chart for acute illness (Department of Health 2004) summarizes the actions for different stages of asthma (Fig. 2).

KEY POINTS

- Asthma is a chronic inflammatory disease affecting the lower airways resulting in bronchoconstriction
- It has a prevalence of 10–23% in England
- Acute asthma causes approximately 1000 deaths in the UK per year
- Asthma should be suspected in any child with an audible wheeze, recurrent cough and breathlessness with acute exacerbations
- Triggers include infection, allergy, airborne chemicals, passive smoking and exercise
- Signs, symptoms and treatment regimes are categorized by age
- Treatment for acute exacerbations will include bronchodilators and steroids ± oxygen and hospital admission

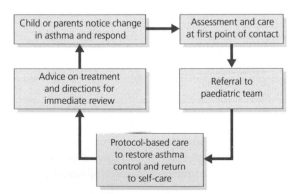

Figure 2 The National Service Framework flow chart for acute illness (Department of Health 2004).

Currie, G.P., Devereux, G.S., Lee, D.K.C. & Ayres, J.G. (2005) Recent developments in asthma management. *BMJ* **330**, 585–589.

Department of Health. (2004) *Asthma exemplar. National Service Framework for Children, Young People and Maternity Services.* http://www.dh.gov.uk/en/ Publicationsandstatistics/Publications/Publications-PolicyAndGuidance/DH_4089205 Accessed on 13 March 2007.

Joint Royal Colleges Ambulance Liaison Committee. (2004) *Recognition of the Seriously Ill Child.* Joint Royal Colleges Ambulance Liaison Committee, London.

National Institute for Health and Clinical Excellence (NICE). (2002) *Inhaler devices for routine treatment of chronic asthma in older children (aged 5–15 years).* Technology Appraisal Guidance No. 38. http://guidance.nice.org/TA38/guidance/pdf/English Accessed on 13 March 2007.

Case 3 A 27-year-old woman with a headache

A 27-year-old woman, who you do not know, attends the surgery. Ewa is Polish and has recently registered with your practice, having immigrated a few months ago. She has attended for a new patient screening appointment a couple of weeks ago, has no past medical history of note and is not on any medication. She attends today complaining of a headache. She is with her husband, Dominik, who is acting as her interpreter as she speaks very little English.

What are the important questions to ask a patient with a headache?

See Box 3.

You need to remember that you will be talking via a translator. Using her husband as a translator is convenient but there are issues with patient confidentiality and using him may alter the history that you will hear (Box 4). Histories via interpreters can be very time-consuming and will also pose problems if you need to carry out an intimate examination.

You ask Ewa whether she is happy for Dominik to act as her translator or whether she would prefer a translator who would speak to them via a telephone. She opts for her husband.

Ewa says that she has always had occasional headaches but 3 or 4 months ago they started occurring daily. She occasionally wakes with a headache and they can last most of the day. They are bilateral, pulsating in nature when they are at their worst and ease to a mild ache behind her eyes. Once or twice she tried paracetamol and co-codamol which she bought from the chemist, but they did not help much.

She sometimes feels a little sick with the headaches if they are bad, but has no other symptoms. She has not had headaches like this in the past although she was diagnosed with migraines when she was a teenager but they felt different. She has not identified any triggers.

Box 3 Headache history

(After British Association for the Study of Headache 2007.)
- Time questions:
  - How long have they experienced the headache?
  - How often do they have a headache?
  - How long does it last for?
  - Why are they consulting now?
- Character questions:
  - Intensity of pain
  - Nature of pain
  - Site of pain
- Associated symptoms
- Cause questions:
  - Triggers
  - Precipitating or relieving factors
  - Family history
- Response questions:
  - How does it affect their daily activities?
  - What do they take for their headache?
- Are they well between attacks?

Box 4 Language services for non-English speakers

(After Phelan & Parkman 1995.)
- *Bilingual health workers:* ideal but rare
- *Trained interpreters:* maintain a strict code of confidentiality, skilled at interpreting while preserving the content of the interview. This can include telephone interpretation services
- *Friends or relatives:* readily available, knowledgeable about patient's problems, presence can be reassuring but on the other hand may hinder the patient and so they could fail to disclose information. They also could deliberately alter the information given
- *Untrained volunteers:* the main concern is confidentiality

Table 5 Differential diagnosis of headache. [After Hopcroft & Forte 1999.]

Common	Rare
Tension headache	Cluster headache
Migraine	Trigeminal neuralgia
Eye strain	Primary angle-closure glaucoma
Dehydration	Carbon monoxide poisoning
Medication overuse headache	Subarachnoid or other intracranial bleed
Cervicogenic (arising from the neck)	Temporal arteritis
Sinusitis	Meningitis/encephalitis Brain tumour Idiopathic benign intracranial hypertension Severe hypertension

What are the different causes of headache?
See Table 5.

What are the two most likely diagnoses in this case?
- Chronic tension-type headache
- Medication overuse headache

When do patients get medication overuse headache? Is this therefore likely to be the cause of Ewa's headache?
Patients are at risk if they have been using analgesics or triptans for more than 17 days a month. Codeine-based products are a particular problem (Fuller & Kaye 2007). As Ewa has only used analgesics occasionally this is an unlikely cause.

What is the most important question that has not been covered and why is it important?
What is Ewa worried that it might be? Exploring and addressing the patient's fears in a consultation about headache is extremely important as patients are often worried about the possibility of a brain tumour. Another common worry is hypertension.

She starts crying and looks very upset when you ask this. She says that she is worried that she might have a brain tumour. She explains that she went to see her previous doctor in Poland when she visited home recently and he arranged a brain scan. This made her think that there must be something seriously wrong. Her doctor was on holiday when she needed to return to England and so she never found out the result. She hands you a packet of computed tomography (CT) films. You look in vain for a report.

What are the red flag symptoms of headache that you need to think about which could indicate serious pathology?

> **!RED FLAG**
>
> Symptoms for headache (Fuller & Kaye 2007; NGC 2006). Dangerous headaches include those called first and worst (single and of sudden onset)
> - Progressive headaches over weeks/months (intracranial lesion)
> - Sudden explosive headache 'like a blow to the head' (subarachnoid)
> - Pregnant woman in third trimester (eclampsia)
> - New and increasing headache on waking, increased by stooping or straining (raised intracranial pressure)
> - New headache in those over 50 years old (temporal artertitis)
> - Associated fever (infection)
> - Seizures (intracranial lesion)

Does she have any of these symptoms?
She does not present with any of these apart from occasionally waking up with a headache but this is not new.

What should you do next?
You should complete your own assessment by examining her.

What are the components of a full examination for headache?
See Box 5.

In a well patient in general practice some of these components are not necessary.

> **Box 5 Headache examination**
>
> NGC (2006).
> - Vital signs
> - *Neurological examination:* Glasgow Coma Score, opthalmological, cranial nerves, peripheral nervous system
> - *Extracranial structures:* carotid arteries, sinuses, temporal arteries, cervical examination

She has a pulse rate of 82 beats/min, BP of 112/78 mmHg, normal central and peripheral nervous system examination, no tenderness over the sinuses or temporal arteries. Cervical spine is non-tender with full range of movement. Ewa has 6/6 vision, in both eyes, measured using a Snellen chart.

Does your assessment make you think that the patient should have a brain scan (this would usually need to be accessed via a neurologist)?

You do not have a high index of suspicion of an intracranial lesion in this patient and so do not think that a scan is necessary. Although a scan can be useful in reducing patient's fears, one study found that patients who were offered a scan were less anxious at 3 months but there was no difference at 1 year (Howard *et al.* 2005).

This leaves you in a dilemma as the patient has already had a scan, which you do not feel was indicated, and you do not have a report for it.

What are your possible courses of action?

- Ask the patient to contact her doctor in Poland to ask for a summary of their consultation and for a report of the CT scan
- Ask a friendly local radiologist if they would be prepared to report on the CT scan
- Refer the patient to a neurologist, informing them of your predicament
- Trust your own assessment that the patient does not need a scan and treat her as if she had not been seen in Poland

Is it ethical to get a scan on a patient if there is no indication?

You should not perform unnecessary investigations particularly if it involves radiation exposure. However, if questions are raised from an investigation that has previously been performed, even if not by you, then you should follow it up.

You weigh up the different options and decide that the best action is to ask the couple to contact their doctor in Poland. They promise to do this but the husband calls you the following week to say that he cannot get hold of the doctor.

You therefore decide to call a radiology colleague at the local hospital and explain the case. She agrees to look at the scan but warns you that the patient may need to be rescanned if the images are not clear or if they show any indication of pathology.

The CT scan is reported as normal.

What is the most likely diagnosis?

The most likely diagnosis is tension-type headache.

What do you tell the patient?

Reassurance is the most important part of managing this case. You should tell the couple that the scan that was performed in Poland has been reported as normal and that you think that the diagnosis is tension headache.

Dominik immediately responds to this by asking if you think that Ewa is stressed.

You respond by saying that tension headaches can be caused by stress and ask if she thinks that this is the cause. She explains that she is missing her friends and family in Poland and that she has not settled well in the UK. Dominik adds that they are making much more money here than they did at home and so even though she is not happy it would be better if they could stay.

What are the treatment options for tension-type headache?

See Box 6.

> **Box 6 Treatment of tension-type headache**
>
> (After British Association for the Study of Headaches 2007.)
> - Exercise: tension-type headache is more common in sedentary people
> - Physiotherapy if there is a musculoskeletal problem
> - Relaxation therapy and cognitive training
> - Removal of stressors
> - Medication: including anti-inflammatories, amitriptyline or paracetamol (although the latter is less effective)

You say that you want to discuss possible treatments but that her distress is probably contributing to the headaches. Ewa says that she has heard that yoga can help and asks if she could try this first as she does not want any form of talking therapy or drugs. You agree with this and say that you would

like to follow her up in a month. You stress to her that she should return sooner if her symptoms get any worse.

Outcome. Ewa and her husband move out of the practice area within a couple of months without returning to see you. You are left not knowing whether her symptoms improved.

CASE REVIEW

Headaches are one of the most common reasons for attending the GP, with the lifetime prevalence being 96%. Most are benign and tension-type headaches are the most common (lifetime prevalence of 30–78%; Fuller & Kaye 2007). Chronic tension-type headaches are more prevalent in women and there is often a family history. Symptoms can start at younger than 10 years of age and the prevalence declines with age (Silver 2007).

As with all patients with headache, this case highlighted the importance of exploring the patient's ideas and concerns. If you do not address these, a management plan that is satisfactory to both the patient and the doctor cannot be reached.

Underlying contributory factors are extremely important in tension-type headache and effective treatment relies on their identification and treatment. Chronic tension headache can be refractory and these patients often end up in chronic pain management clinics. Some patients may use alternative therapies such as acupuncture or homeopathy but both of these are of unknown effectiveness (British Association for the Study of Headaches 2007).

We have many patients from all over the world coming from different systems of health care, often from countries where many unnecessary investigations are carried out giving rise to high patient expectations. Every effort should be made to understand their culture and expectations so that they can be dealt with appropriately but this can be very difficult.

Dealing with patients who move in and out of your practice area can be frustrating for you as a medical practitioner. However, you should remember that these individuals often have poor medical management, particularly as they get lost to follow-up. If they are non-English speakers this will also put them at a disadvantage and so every effort should be made to optimize their care while they are with your practice.

KEY POINTS

- Headaches have a lifetime prevalence of 96%
- They are many causes, most are benign but patients often worry about sinister causes
- History should include questions about time, character, cause, response, associated symptoms and whether the patient is well between attacks
- Examination could include vital signs, neurological examination and extracranial structures: carotid
arteries, sinuses, temporal arteries, cervical examination
- Medication overuse should always be considered in those with chronic headache
- Treatment of tension-type headache includes identification of precipitants, reassurance, exercise, physiotherapy, relaxation therapy, cognitive training and medication

References

British Association for the Study of Headaches. (2007) *Guidelines for all healthcare professionals in the diagnosis and management of migraine, tension-type, cluster and medication-overuse headache.* www.bash. org.uk Accessed on 5 May 2007.

Fuller, G. & Kaye, C. (2007) Headaches: masterclass for GPs. *BMJ* **334**, 254–256.

Hopcroft, K. & Forte, V. (1999) *Symptom Sorter.* Radcliffe Medical Press, Abingdon.

Howard, L., Wessely, S., Leese, M., Page, L., McCrone, P., Husain, K., *et al.* (2005) Are investigations anxiolytic or anxiogenic? A randomised controlled trial of neuroimaging to provide reassurance in chronic daily headache. *Journal of Neurology, Neurosurgery and Psychiatry* **76**, 1558–1564.

National Guideline Clearinghouse (NGC). (2006) *Diagnosis and treatment of headache.* Institute for Clinical Systems Improvement. www.guideline.gov Accessed on 5 May 2007.

Phelan, M. & Parkman, S. (1995) How to do it: work with an interpreter. *BMJ* **311**, 555–557.

Silver, N. (2007) Headache (chronic tension-type) clinical evidence. *BMJ* http://0-www.clinicalevidence.com Accessed on 4 June 2007.

A 76-year-old man who has been in hospital

You are asked to carry out a home visit to Mr Richards, a 76-year-old West Indian man who joined your practice a few months ago and whom you have never met. His daughter, Mrs Grant, has rung to say that her father has recently been discharged from hospital following a stroke. She would like a visit as soon as possible.

Unfortunately, the hospital discharge letter has not arrived yet. Mr Richards' previous medical notes show that he was diagnosed with high blood pressure 8 years ago and he has been taking atenolol 50 mg o.d. and bendroflumethiazide 2.5 mg o.d. He is a non-smoker and lives alone. There is no information regarding a recent hospital admission and he last saw his previous GP 10 months ago.

What should you do first?

Phone Mrs Grant to confirm that you are coming to see her father and to ask for more information about what has happened to him.

What will you need in your doctor's bag?

• Sphygmomanometer and stethoscope
• Urine specimen bottle and dipstick (urinary infections are common in the elderly and you want to exclude proteinuria and/or glycosuria)

If this was an acute situation, you might want to take a reflex hammer and equipment for testing cranial nerves. However, the diagnosis of a stroke has already been made so your role will be more to do with his rehabilitation and prevention of further strokes in the future.

When you speak to Mrs Grant, she tells you that her father has been in hospital for 7 weeks and was discharged home yesterday. She is worried that he will not be able to cope on his own and may fall. She thinks the hospital said they would contact the district nurses, but no-one has been yet. She is now at work but arranges to meet you at Mr. Richards' flat in 20 min.

The home visit

At the flat, Mrs Grant shows you into a cluttered front room with piles of papers and magazines on the floor and every available surface. Mr Richards is sitting in an armchair in front of an electric heater, which is on full blast. There is a strong smell of urine.

You introduce yourself and try to shake Mr Richards' right hand but he cannot return your grip. He smiles lopsidedly and says 'Hallo Doc' in a slurred tone. Mrs Grant bursts into tears and rocks back and forth on the sofa.

What should you do next?

• Reassure Mrs Grant that you will do everything you can to help her father
• Suggest that she goes and makes a cup of tea while you examine Mr Richards. (This will be less distracting for you and gives her a practical task to do which may help her regain control)
• Find out from Mr Richards how he is feeling, if he has any urinary symptoms and what he wants for the future

Mr Richards gives you a copy of the handwritten hospital discharge letter which confirms a left-sided cerebrovascular accident (CVA). You notice that some of his medications have been changed:

Bendroflumethiazide 2.5 mg o.d.
Diltiazem SR 240 mg o.d.
Aspirin EC 75 mg o.d.
Dipyridamole MR 200 mg b.i.d.
Metformin 500 mg t.i.d.
Paracetamol 500 mg p.r.n.
Simvastatin 40 mg nocte

What does this list tell you about the sort of stroke that Mr Richards has had and any other diagnoses that have been made?

Mr Richards must have had an atherothrombotic or embolic stroke causing cerebral occlusion, rather than a haemorrhagic stroke as he has been put on aspirin and dipyridamole antiplatelet therapy to prevent further incidents and simvastatin to lower lipid levels. He has also been started on a biguanide (metformin), suggesting that a diagnosis of diabetes was made. This has not been mentioned in the hospital letter.

Why might the medicines for high blood pressure have been changed?

Evidence suggests that certain drugs (β-blockers and angiotensin converting enzyme (ACE) inhibitors) are less effective in people of Afro-Carribean origin, so calcium channel blockers and thiazides are recommended (NICE 2006, Williams *et al.* 2004). You notice that diltiazem, a calcium channel blocker has been added to his medication.

What further information do you need?

You have already observed a great deal. Mr Richards has obvious right facial weakness and his speech and right hand have been affected by the stroke. Is his right leg also weak? Can he understand everything you say to him? Is he depressed, a common problem in anyone who has had a CVA. Does he drink any alcohol? If so, how much? (Excessive alcohol predisposes to both ischaemic and haemorrhagic stroke.) How is his arthritis?
• Check Mr Richards' pulse for arrythmias (a common cause of embolic stroke)
• Measure his blood pressure
• Dipstick a urine sample for leucocytes, nitrites, sugar and protein

You should also assess how mobile he is and if he can manage going to the toilet on his own. Is he able to make himself a hot drink and cook a meal? The hospital should have arranged these latter assessments before sending him home, but in this case it is not clear whether this has happened.

Mr Richards understands everything you ask him although he is limited to 'Yes' and 'No' answers. Mrs Grant tells you that the occupational therapist and physiotherapist did do some home visits with Mr Richards. before he left hospital

and he has been given a tripod walking stick, a rail by the toilet and a shelf to fit over the bath.

Mr Richards seems to be feeling well and in good spirits. You note that he is quite overweight. He has no urinary symptoms. He drinks alcohol occasionally. He is aware that he has diabetes but is not able to carry out blood or urine tests himself. He is getting some pain in his left hip from the arthritis, but the paracetamol helps.

His pulse is 80 beats/min regular and BP 148/84 mmHg sitting. He is able to get up out of his chair with difficulty and walk with the stick, but he drags his right foot. He says he can make himself a cup of tea, but cooking is going to be difficult. He is quite clear that he wants to stay in his own home and not go into residential care.

What are the main hazards for Mr Richards' health?

• Further strokes – chances minimized by good control of blood pressure (<130/80 mmHg) (British Hypertension Guidelines 2004)
• Falls because of poor mobility and not helped by the clutter in the flat
• Worsening diabetes – medication and diet crucial
• Failing to take his medications – may be a memory problem (common after a stroke) or the difficulty in opening containers and taking several different preparations
• Fire risk – particularly with all the papers around

Mrs Grant is still upset and mutters something about her father not being ready to come home and the Ward Sister wanting to clear the beds. She says she has a family of her own to look after, a full-time job and she cannot be 'coming in and out to my Dad all the time'. She implies that you should sort things out now.

How should you respond to this situation?

You should not be drawn into blaming the hospital or staff as this would be unprofessional and it is not clear how this situation has arisen. Mrs Grant is obviously anxious about her father and this may make her angry or unreasonable. You explain that you will try to organize as much help as you can for Mr Richards, but this will involve several telephone calls from the surgery. You take her mobile telephone number and ask if there is any chance that she or her brother might stay with Mr Richards tonight while you sort things out.

What agencies should you contact for further help?

- District nurses – can help with testing his blood sugar regularly and assisting with bathing, dressing, etc.
- Social Services to arrange Meals on Wheels
- Pharmacist to provide a dosette box with all the medications loaded on a weekly basis
- Consider referral to community physiotherapy and/or speech therapy, but this will depend on what the hospital has already arranged

Is there any support you can offer Mrs Grant?

You might suggest she gets in touch with the Stroke Association which offers practical advice and organizes local support groups in some areas for patients and their carers (Stroke Association Tel: 0845 30 33 100 http://www.stroke.org.uk).

Mr Richards is unable to provide a urine sample so you leave the specimen bottle with him and ask Mrs Grant to drop it in to the surgery tomorrow morning. You explain to Mr Richards that you are concerned about his ability to manage on his own at home but that you will organize help for him as soon as you can.

Is there anyone else you should talk to about Mr Richards?

Contact the ward where Mr Richards was a patient and talk to the Sister to find out what help has already been put in place and what the follow-up arrangements are.

Discuss Mr Richards' case with your colleague(s) who run the diabetic clinic at the practice and make him an appointment to be seen there in a few months time.

Back at the surgery

It takes several attempts to get through to the ward, but when you speak to the Sister, she confirms that the assessment by the occupational therapist and physiotherapist was that Mr Richards can cope on his own at home. The district nurses have been contacted and are due to visit tomorrow morning. He will be seen in outpatients in 6 weeks. No further hospital rehabilitation has been planned.

What should you do next?

- Ring the district nurses to confirm that they have received the referral and are planning to visit tomorrow
- Contact the other agencies as suggested above

- Ring Mrs Grant to inform her about these arrangements and to remind her to bring in the urine sample
- Arrange to see Mr Richards again in 1 week to recheck his blood pressure and see how he is doing

Mrs Grant tells you that her brother has agreed to stay tonight with Mr Richards. She still sounds upset but thanks you for trying to help.

What should you enter in Mr Richards' medical notes?

- Document your findings at the home visit
- List the agencies you have contacted so far
- Update his medication list and add a review date of 3 months' time
- Add the diagnoses of stroke and diabetes to his record
- Print out microbiology form to send with the urine sample tomorrow

You should also enter Mr Richards' wishes to stay at home. If Mrs Grant is not a patient at the practice, you should add her contact details as primary carer.

In the long term

Looking after Mr Richards in the community is going to involve several different agencies. It would be a good idea to arrange a meeting between all these people in a few weeks time so everyone is aware of who is involved in his care and the long-term rehabilitation plan.

The issue of the clutter in the flat is a difficult one to tackle at this early stage. If you feel he is at severe risk of falling and/or fire because of the state of the flat, you could mention this to Mrs Grant and Mr Richards next time you visit. Otherwise, you could leave raising the issue until you have got to know them better and established a good relationship with them. Similarly, the problem of Mr Richards' weight will affect his mobility and diabetes. You may want to suggest a low fat, low salt diet and possibly refer him to a dietitian to help with weight loss in the long run.

References and further reading

National Institute for Health and Clinical Excellence (NICE). (2006) *Hypertension: management of hypertension in adults in primary care*. Clinical guideline. http://www.nice.org.uk Accessed on 15 July 2007.

Royal College of Physicians. (2004) *National Clinical Guidelines for Stroke*, 2nd edn. Available from http://www.rcplondon.ac.uk Accessed on 15 July 2007.

CASE REVIEW

Stroke is the most common cause of adult disability in the UK and often devastating for the patient and their family. As the GP looking after a patient who has experienced such an event, treatment of coexisting conditions is crucial, both in maintaining independence and mobility and in preventing further strokes. Mr Richards presents a complex but common case scenario in that he has several risk factors (diabetes, hypertension, overweight and poor living conditions). Depression and memory impairment may be a problem after a stroke and need careful and regular monitoring.

If Mr Richards is going to be able to remain at home, his daughter, Mrs Grant, is going to need a lot of support as well and be actively involved in decisions about his care. It may be that her brother can also play a more active part. Some support may come from the voluntary sector as well as Social Services, nursing and physiotherapy agencies. It

may be that she can claim Attendance Allowance to help with his care. Coordination of everyone involved in Mr Richards' rehabilitation is crucial to the success of his wish to stay at home. The local pharmacist should also be informed about the change to his medication and a weekly dosette box may well help Mr Richards to remember to take his tablets regularly. Finally, communication between secondary and primary care and meticulous recording of diagnoses is part of good patient care. In this case, it was not clear from the hospital discharge letter what assessments and arrangements had been made for Mr Richards prior to his leaving the ward.

NICE guidelines recommend a combination of modified release dipyridamole and low dose aspirin for anyone who has had an ischaemic stroke or transient ischaemic attack (TIA) for a period of 2 years from the most recent event (NICE 2006).

KEY POINTS

- Stroke is the most common cause of adult disability in the UK (Simon *et al.* 2005)
- Half of all strokes occur in people over the age of 70 years
- Organized, specialist inpatient care, such as that provided in a stroke unit, is associated with improved outcomes (Young & Forster 2007)
- In England, less that half of patients admitted with a stroke are treated on stroke units

- Risk factors for stroke include: raised blood pressure, diabetes, age, smoking, obesity, alcohol, previous stroke, TIAs or myocardial infarction, atrial fibrillation and low physical activity
- Around 70% of strokes are thromboembolic and 19% haemorrhagic

Scottish Intercollegiate Guidelines Network (SIGN). (2006) *Management of patients with stroke, rehabilitation, prevention and management of complications and discharge planning.* http://www.sign.ac.uk Accessed on 15 July 2007.

Simon, C., Everitt, H. & Kendrick, T. (2005) *Oxford Handbook of General Practice,* 2nd edn. Oxford University Press, Oxford.

Williams, B., Poulter, N.R., Brown, M.J., Davis, M., McInnes, G.T., Potter, J.P., *et al.* (2004) The BHS Guidelines Working Party. *British Hypertension Society Guidelines for Hypertension Management, 2004, BHS IV: Summary. BMJ* **328**, 634–640. http://www.bhsoc.org Accessed on 15 July 2007.

Young, J. & Forster, A. (2007) Rehabilitation after stroke. *BMJ* **334**, 86–90.

Case 5   A 23-year-old man with a red eye

Mr Ndovu is a 23-year-old African man from Zimbabwe who has recently registered with your practice. You have met him once before when he came with a chest infection and was treated with antibiotics. Now he comes in complaining that his right eye is painful, watering and red. This has been going on for about 2 days and getting worse.

What causes of a red eye can you think of?
- *Conjunctivitis:* purulent discharge usually present
- *Blepharitis:* inflammation of the lids
- *Keratitis:* corneal problem
- *Iritis:* also known as anterior uveitis
- *Episcleritis:* inflammation of the membrane covering the sclera of the eye, red and diffuse with no discharge and not much pain
- *Acute glaucoma:* severe pain, eye cloudy and vision impaired, usually in those aged over 50 years
- *Corneal abrasion:* history of trauma
- *Subconjunctival haemorrhage:* red eye with no discomfort, often a discrete spot
- *Inflamed pterygium:* fleshy growth on the surface of the eye in the elderly

What questions do you need to ask him?
- Has he been doing anything that might have led to an injury to the eye?
- What is his job?
- Is his vision affected?
- Is the eye sticky?
- Is he allergic to anything?
- How bad is the pain?
- Does he wear contact lenses?

- Has he had this before?
- Has he tried any treatment himself?

Mr Ndovu tells you that he works in a care home looking after elderly patients. He has not suffered any injuries to the eye. He has no known allergies. The right eye is very painful and he is having trouble seeing properly out of it. He does not wear contact lenses. There has not been any discharge from the eye and he has not had this before. He went to the chemist who gave him some eye drops but they have not helped.

You remember that occasionally a painful red eye is associated with Reiter's syndrome. What other questions are relevant if you suspect this condition?
- Has he had any recent flu-like illnesses?
- Has he had any aching or stiffness in his joints (wrists, fingers, knees and ankles)?
- Has he noticed any pain on urination and/or a penile discharge?
- Has he had any sores in the mouth or on the genitals?

Mr Ndovu answers 'no' to all of these questions. He is having trouble keeping his right eye open while he talks to you and covers it with his hand.

Why do his symptoms not sound like conjunctivitis? (the most common cause of red eye seen in general practice)
He has pain, rather than just discomfort and there is no history of sticky eye.

What Red Flag symptoms and signs would alert you to the fact that this might be a serious ocular problem and warrant urgent referral?

!RED FLAG

- Pain in the eye
- Photophobia
- Reduced visual acuity
- Ciliary flush (ring of red or violet around the cornea)
- Corneal oedema or opacities
- Corneal epithelial disruption (only visible on staining the eye)
- Difference in size or shape between the pupils on normal and affected eyes

All of the above 'Red flags' can signal a serious eye problem that might lead to permanent loss of vision if not investigated and treated by a specialist.

What examination should you do?

You should first inspect and compare both Mr Ndovu's eyes. Is there a difference in size of the pupils? (A dilated pupil suggests glaucoma whereas a constricted pupil suggests iritis.) Where is the right eye red? Is there any obvious discharge?

It is often easier to look at the eye and fundus in subdued lighting so you warn Mr Ndovu that you are going to switch off the lights in the room or draw the curtains or blinds.

Using the ophthalmoscope:
- Examine the cornea
- Examine the anterior chamber (space between the cornea and the iris)
- Inspect the iris, conjunctiva and fundus

You should now turn the lights back on. Measure the visual acuity in both eyes, checking first to see if he usually wears glasses and asking him to put these on before you ask him to read the Snellen chart.

Mr Ndovu's right eyelids are inflamed and the eye appears red mainly around the cornea, and there is some watering but no discharge. The iris appears normal and there is no pus visible in the anterior chamber. The pupils are equal in size and react to light. You are not sure if the cornea has some dull patches which could be opacities. The fundus appears normal but it is difficult to visualize it adequately as he finds the light painful.

He is tender in the pre-auricular region on the right side. Mr Ndovu does not wear glasses and his visual acuity is 6/6 in the left eye and 6/18 in the right.

What other investigation is useful at this stage?

Staining the eye with fluorescein drops and then examining the cornea using a cobalt blue light (which should be available on the ophthalmoscope). A disruption to the corneal epithelium will show up as green.

When you look at Mr Ndovu's eye again after putting in the fluorescein eyedrops, you can see a definite green lesion on the cornea (Plate 1, facing p. 56).

What is your diagnosis and what are you going to do next?

Mr Nduvo has keratitis (inflammation of the cornea) of unknown origin. This is a serious condition that can lead to scarring and loss of vision. His visual acuity is already less in the right eye than the left (although this could be normal for him). An urgent referral to the ophthalmology clinic is necessary so the cause can be diagnosed and treated.

What are the possible causes of keratitis?

- Infectious (amoebic, bacterial, and fungal, which are all more common in contact lens wearers. Viral – may be caused by herpes simplex or zoster) leading to ulceration
- Photokeratitis caused by intense ultraviolet radiation (snow blindness or welder's arc eye)
- Severe allergic response leading to corneal inflammation and ulceration
- Dry eyes from disorders of the eyelids or diminished ability to make tears
- Vitamin A deficiency

Should you prescribe any treatment?

No – you do not know exactly what you are treating. *Steroid drops should never be prescribed for an undiagnosed red eye.*

What do you say to Mr Ndovu about your findings?

You explain to him that you have found severe inflammation in the outer part of the right eye and are going to refer him urgently to see an eye specialist at the hospital for treatment.

Mr Ndovu is very worried that he is going to go blind. He asks you if he will lose the sight in his eye.

If this is the first episode of keratitis and he is treated quickly and appropriately, there is a good chance that his vision will not be affected permanently. You can reassure him that it is likely his right eye will recover completely, but it does depend on the diagnosis and cause of the keratitis, as well as his response to the treatment.

What is likely to happen to him at the hospital?

At the hospital, they will examine his eyes with a slit lamp, measure the pressure in each eye, take swabs and then treat him with eye drops (antibiotic, antiviral or antifungal depending on the diagnosis).

What follow-up will you arrange?

You suggest he comes back to see you in a few days so you can make sure his symptoms are improving and he is managing to take the prescribed treatment. You write an urgent referral letter to the ophthalmologist, give it to Mr Ndovu and ring up whoever is on call for eye emergencies at the hospital to arrange for him to be seen that day.

Three days later

Mr Ndovu returns with a letter from the ophthalmologist confirming a diagnosis of corneal ulcer caused by a herpes simplex infection (HSV-1) – a dendritic ulcer. He has been prescribed aciclovir cream to apply 5 times a day for 10 days and given another appointment in the eye clinic in 2 weeks time. He has been told to stay off work until then.

He asks you why he has developed this problem and if it is likely to recur?

What do you know about herpes infections and what should you tell him?

You can honestly say that you are not sure why he developed the ulcer now, although there are various trigger factors that are known to reactivate the herpes virus living in the trigeminal ganglion.

What are these factors?

- Stress
- UV light
- Systemic illness
- Fever
- Local trauma
- Cold wind
- Immunosuppression

It is possible that the problem could recur (20% in 2 years and 40% in 5 years, according to Prodigy guidance 2007) in which case he should seek medical help straight away.

It occurs to you that Mr Ndovu comes from a country where there is a high incidence of HIV infection. How might you find out if he has been at risk of being HIV positive?

This is a difficult topic to raise but you can ask if he has any particular worries about his health and find out if he has been unwell at all in the last few years. You might also ask if he has a partner or wife. You could ask if he has ever had a blood transfusion or used intravenous drugs.

Mr Ndovu tells you that he is not married. He has had several girlfriends both in Zimbabwe and in the UK but is not in a permanent relationship at present. He has never had a blood transfusion or used IV drugs. He understands what you are referring to and volunteers that he had a HIV test 6 months ago which was negative.

Should you offer to retest him for HIV?

You should take a full sexual history to see if he might be at risk of HIV infection and/or hepatitis B. Pre-counselling for HIV tests is advisable and in many areas is carried out in the local genitourinary clinic, although increasingly GPs also perform both the testing and counselling themselves.

How long does it take from exposure to HIV for the blood test to show up as positive?

Most people develop detectable HIV antibodies within 6–12 weeks of infection. In very rare cases, it can take up to 6 months (Box 7). It is exceedingly rare for someone to take longer than 6 months to develop antibodies.

It seems that Mr Ndovu might be at risk of HIV because he has had unprotected sex with two women he did not know well in the last 2 months. You suggest that he attends the sexual health clinic for a full sexually transmitted infection (STI) check-up and arranges a repeat HIV test 3 months from his last sexual encounter. You offer to see him again when he has the results of these tests in a few weeks time.

Box 7 HIV testing

Getting tested earlier than 3 months may result in an unclear test result, as an infected person may not yet have developed antibodies to HIV. The time between infection and the development of antibodies is called the window period. In the window period people infected with HIV have no antibodies in their blood that can be detected by an HIV test. However, the person may already have high levels of HIV in their blood, sexual fluids or breast milk. HIV can be passed on to another person during the window period even though an HIV test will not show that you are infected with HIV. So it is best to wait for at least 3 months after the last time you were at risk before taking the test. Some test centres may recommend testing again at 6 months, just to be extra sure.

What other advice will you give him?

You counsel him about safe sex practices and offer him some condoms (some practices keep these in stock and give them out in small quantities). You also give him the details of where the nearest sexual health clinic is situated and how to get in touch with them.

You tell Mr Ndovu that his right eye should go on improving but if the problem recurs he should seek medical help as soon as possible.

Mr Ndovu is satisfied with these arrangements and says he will ring up for an appointment with you shortly. He thanks you for your help and concern.

CASE REVIEW

Conjunctivitis is the most common cause of red eye and accounts for about 35% of all eye complaints seen in general practice. This usually presents with irritation rather than pain in the eye, redness and some clear or purulent discharge, depending on whether it is a viral or bacterial cause. In Mr Ndovu's case, the fact his eye is acutely painful and there is no discharge should alert you to the fact that this is unlikely to be conjunctivitis, but something more serious. Ocular herpes simplex is not something you will see very often in general practice but is the most common infective cause of corneal blindness in high-income countries. According to the Prodigy guidance (2007), it has a prevalence of 1.5 cases per 1000 population with an equal male : female ratio.

Systematic examination of both eyes, including visual acuity and staining with fluorescein drops, is important in the differential diagnosis of a red eye. You should have a low threshold for referral to an ophthalmologist if there is any history of impairment of vision. The specialist (and the patient) will not criticize you for not being able to distinguish between iritis and keratitis as long as you recog-

nize the 'Red flag' situations that need urgent referral. Conditions involving the conjunctivae and eyelids may cause enlargement of the pre-auricular lymph nodes, as in this case.

Complications of herpes simplex keratitis include scarring of the cornea and visual loss, perforated corneal ulcer, secondary bacterial infection, secondary glaucoma and systemic involvement, so it is essential that early diagnosis occurs and treatment is started.

Mr Ndovu's case also raises the issue of his HIV status. Many people from countries where the virus is widespread, such as sub-Saharan Africa, will already have had a blood test but it is important to take a full sexual and drug history to check whether they might be at risk. Other STIs that are relevant include *Chlamydia* and gonorrhoea, both of which can cause eye symptoms. Depending on your expertise and local access to a sexual health clinic, you may want to take urethral swabs for gonorrhoea and send a first pass urine sample for *Chlamydia*. In Mr Ndovu's case, the priority was to refer him to the eye clinic urgently and then to arrange other investigations at the sexual health clinic.

KEY POINTS

- In general practice, 2–5% consultations concern the eye (Manners 1997, quoted in Prodigy guidance)
- Most red eyes in general practice are not painful
- Accurate diagnosis of the cause of a red eye is less important than knowing when to refer on urgently
- Pain in the eye, reduced visual acuity and photophobia are all indicative of serious eye disease and warrant urgent referral
- Steroid drops should *never* be given for an undiagnosed red eye, reduced visual acuity or when there is a history of a dendritic ulcer because it can lead to permanent scarring and loss of vision
- Keratitis (inflammation of the cornea) is one of the common causes of an uncomfortable red eye
- Acute glaucoma should be considered in anyone over 50 years presenting with an acutely painful red eye
- Impaired immunity may lead to recurrent herpes simplex infections in the eye, skin or mucous membranes

References and further reading

Image of a dendritic ulcer. http://www.opt.indiana.edu/ce/hsk/index.htm Accessed on 17 July 2007.

Prodigy guidance. (2007) *Herpes simplex ocular*. http://www.cks.library.nhs.uk/Herpes_simplex_ocular/In_depth/Backgd_information Accessed on 17 July 2007.

The red eye: diagnostic picture tests. Interactive case history. http://www.bmjlearning.com Accessed on 27 June 2007. A useful website for testing your knowledge and skills in diagnosing causes of red eye.

Case 6 A 5-year-old child with earache

Abby is a 5-year-old girl who is frequently brought to the surgery with minor illnesses. She last attended with her mother a couple of days ago with a mild fever and runny nose. This was diagnosed as a mild upper respiratory tract infection and the mother was advised to treat her symptomatically with paediatric paracetamol or ibuprofen.

Abby has been brought back today by her grandmother, who often looks after her after school while her mother is at work. She is apparently still unwell and is pulling at her ear. The grandmother says that they think that it is an ear infection and that she wants antibiotics for her. Abby looks well on walking into your room.

What would be your immediate thoughts about seeing Abby again so soon?

• Irritation that the family have had to return despite being at the surgery 2 days ago. What has changed? The clinical situation or other factors that impact on the management of the disease and the family's ability to cope?
• Concern that the grandmother has attended with a definite agenda that may or may not be an appropriate treatment plan
• Is this attendance because of concern from the mother or grandmother?

The grandmother is concerned that Abby has an ear infection, what are the symptoms of otitis media?

See Box 8.

> **Box 8 Otitis media presents rapidly with**
>
> SIGN (2003).
> • Earache is the single most important symptom
> • Pulling or tugging at the ears
> • Associated systemic symptoms (e.g. fever, irritability)
> • It may be preceded by upper respiratory symptoms
> Typical symptoms can resolve if the tympanic membrane perforates.

What initial questions do you need to ask?

Remember, Abby will be able to answer some of the questions herself:
• *Is Abby demonstrating any symptoms different from a couple of days ago?*
• *Has she had earache?*
• *Has she been complaining of any other symptoms, for instance sore throat?*
• *How has Abby been eating, sleeping?*

> *She has been pulling at her ear and last time this happened she got better with antibiotics. Abby says that her left ear hurts but has no other symptoms. She has been eating and sleeping normally. The grandmother says that she thinks that she has an ear infection and repeats her request for antibiotics as she cannot cope with Abby when she is ill.*

What is the differential diagnosis?

• Upper respiratory tract infection
• Acute otitis media
• Acute otitis externa
• Chronic suppurative otitis media with effusion

What further sources of information do you have to help you to decide on Abby's clinical condition?

You need to carry out a physical examination to complete your assessment.

What examination should you perform?

• General state of alertness, interactivity, distress
• Hydration
• Colour
• Temperature, but remember this can cause distress in this age group particularly if performed with a tympanic thermometer in a child with earache and it can be unreliable because of the size of the ear canal

• Circulatory assessment including peripheral circulation (only necessary if the child is unwell)
• Respiratory exam
• Ear, nose and throat (ENT) exam looking particularly for a red bulging drum that would indicate a middle ear infection with or without effusion

Remember that most of this examination could be carried out with Abby on her grandmother's knee where she should be at her ease.

> Abby is alert and playful. She is well hydrated and of normal colour. She screams when you approach her with the tympanic thermometer and so you abandon this part of the examination. You next approach her with the auroscope and get a glimpse of both eardrums. The left looks pink but not bulging, the right is normal. There is no discharge. You are not able to get a look at her throat as she is becoming fidgety as she wants to get back to playing on the floor. Her nose is running (clear discharge).

What diagnosis do you make and what treatment would you give her?

Abby appears to have mild acute otitis media but she is well and so her condition does not warrant antibiotics. In about 80% of cases of otitis media it will resolve without antibiotics (O'Neil *et al.* 2006).

When would you give antibiotics in otitis media and what would you give?

See Box 9.

Box 9 Antibiotics in otitis media can be given

BNF for Children (2006).
• If symptoms do not improve after 72 h
• If deterioration occurs
• If the patient is aged under 2 years
• If the patient is immunocompromised
  The first line agent is amoxicillin or erythromycin (if penicillin allergic, for 5 days). If no improvement after 48 h then consider co-amoxiclav. If perforation occurs most children will recover without need for antibacterial agents

---

> You inform the grandmother that it would be better if antibiotics are not used on this occasion because they are

unlikely to cause any reduction in symptoms and could also lead to side-effects including diarrhoea. You reinforce that she should be treated symptomatically with paracetamol or ibuprofen in the appropriate dose for her age and weight.

Is this the end of the consultation?

You should encourage the grandmother to contact the surgery if Abby's condition deteriorates. You should also start to empower the family on how to cope with minor illnesses. This consultation could also be a cry for help from the grandmother. Is she having difficulty coping with Abby? You could explore this further with the family and the health visitor.

What are the options for the management of minor illnesses that you could advise them to use in the future?

See Box 10.

Box 10 Options for management of minor illnesses

(After Porteous *et al.* 2007.)
• Make an appointment with the GP
• Make an appointment to see the practice nurse or nurse practitioner
• Ask for advice from a pharmacist
• Seek advice from a complementary therapist
• Call for information from NHS Direct
• Deal with symptoms yourself with advice from other family members and friends
• Do nothing about the symptoms
• Written material (e.g. *Birth to Five*, which is a book provided by the Department of Health to all parents)

The aim is to empower the family but not to scare them into not contacting the surgery if it is appropriate.

> The grandmother is not happy with this and says that Abby's mother will be very angry if she goes home without a prescription as she is unable to take any time off her job to look after Abby if she is ill. She has recently started work in a factory and has already been disciplined for taking a day off to look after her daughter. As the sole breadwinner at home she cannot afford to lose her job.

What are your options?

- Stand firm and refuse to issue them
- Offer a second opinion with another colleague
- Give the prescription
- Offer a delayed script

As immediate antibiotics are rarely indicated, one option for treatment is to suggest to parents the use of delayed antibiotics. In other words, the parents can collect the script at 72 h at their discretion. This strategy can reduce antibiotic use by 76% as only 24% collected the script (Little *et al.* 2001).

You opt for the delayed script and the grandmother seems reasonably happy after this difficult consultation.

Should you arrange to follow-up otitis media?

The natural history of acute otitis media is that it normally resolves spontaneously and complications are rare so it does not routinely need to be followed up (Box 11).

Box 11 Indications for follow-up for otitis media

1 To visualize the drum if the ear is discharging
2 If an effusion is present. Rarely, incomplete resolution occurs with development of a long-standing effusion (SIGN 2003). Glue ear or middle ear effusion can occur transiently in most children without symptoms. Those that persist can cause problems with speech and language development and so should be referred (Silva et al. 1982)
3 Referral to an ENT specialist should be considered with persistent problems

---

There is no indication to arrange a follow-up appointment in this case.

Abby's condition resolves without the need for the antibiotics and without complication. She is brought to the surgery again within a few weeks with a mild sore throat, this time by her mother.

How should you handle this?

It should be handled like any other consultation. You should not skip parts because you feel that you have been through it all before as you may miss an important diagnosis or a chance to educate the family.

- History
- Examination
- Negotiated management plan
- Parental education

You could also use this as an opportunity to ask about how the family copes with Abby's care while the mother is working.

After taking a history and examining her, a mild upper respiratory tract infection is again diagnosed. They are reassured and a management plan is discussed.

The family will only change in its ability to cope with minor illnesses over a period of time as they slowly gain in confidence.

The mother does not want to discuss Abby's care with you. You offer follow-up with the health visitor and contact her to make her aware of the recent consultations and ask her to contact the family to offer further advice and support.

Outcome. Abby's attendances at the surgery gradually become less frequent and the family still seem happy to consult you with their problems despite your different opinions with her management in the past.

CASE REVIEW

Otitis media is the generic term for middle ear infection and it can occur with or without symptoms. It can occur in acute or chronic states. A total of 75% of all cases of acute otitis media occur in children under 10 years old and one in four children will have an episode during these years. The peak incidence is 3–6 years (SIGN 2003).

Consultations where the patient or parents and the doctor have differing agendas can be difficult to handle and time-consuming. It is important that all management plans are still negotiated and that the GP responds to the concerns of the family. Failure to do this will result in poor compliance and re-attendance with another doctor.

GPs often get into a debate with parents about whether or not their child should be prescribed antibiotics. The evidence base behind not giving antibiotics has increased over the last few years and so most GPs are prescribing less than they did in the past (Box 12).

> ### Box 12 Evidence base for not using antibiotics routinely in otitis media
>
> **1** Many infections are viral and most uncomplicated cases resolve without antibiotics (*BNF for Children* 2006). One meta-analysis has shown that antibiotics do not influence resolution of pain within 24 h of presentation (Del Mar *et al.* 1997)
>
> **2** In cases without fever and vomiting a poor outcome is unlikely (Little *et al.* 2002). Specifically, antibiotics have no influence on recurrence or deafness and they increase the incidence of diarrhoea, vomiting and rashes (Del Mar *et al.* 1997; Glasziou *et al.* 2004)
>
> **3** Number needed to treat: approximately 15 children would need to be given a broad-spectrum antibiotic rather than no antibiotic to prevent one child having pain after 2 days (Glasziou *et al.* 2004)

> ### KEY POINTS
>
> - One in four children under 10 years will have an episode of acute otitis media
> - Symptoms include:
>   - pulling or tugging at the ears
>   - associated systemic symptoms (e.g. fever, irritability)
>   - earache is the single most important symptom
>   - it may be preceded by upper respiratory symptoms
> - Antibiotics are rarely indicated
> - Analgesics will help reduce symptoms
> - A delayed script is one option to reduce antibiotic use
> - The natural history is that it normally resolves spontaneously
> - Glue ear can occur transiently but if it persists it can cause problems so should be referred

References

British National Formulary for Children. (2006) Royal Pharmaceutical Society of Great Britain. RPS Publishing and BMJ Publishing Group, London.

Del Mar, C.B., Glasziou, P.P. & Hayern, M. (1997) Are antibiotics indicated as initial treatment for children with acute otitis media? A meta-analysis. *BMJ* **314**, 1526–1529.

Glasziou, P.P., Del Mar, C.B., Sanders, S.L. & Hayem, M. (2004) Antibiotics for acute otitis media in children. *Cochrane Database of Systematic Reviews* Issue 1. Art No.: CD000219. DOI:10.1002/14651858.CD000219.pub2.

Little, P., Gould, C., Williamson, I., Moore, M., Warner, G. & Dunleavey, J. (2001) Pragmatic randomised controlled trial of two prescribing strategies for childhood acute otitis media. *BMJ* **322**, 336–342.

Little, P., Gould, C., Moore, M., Warner M., Dunleavey, J. & Williamson, I. (2002) Predictors of poor outcome and benefits from antibiotics in children with otitis media: pragmatic randomised trial. *BMJ* **325**, 22.

O'Neill, P., Roberts, T. & Bradley-Stevenson, C. (2006) Otitis media in children (acute). *Clinical Evidence* British Medical Journal Publishing Group. www.clinicalevidence.com Accessed on 2 March 2007.

Porteous, T., Ryan, M., Bond, C.M. & Hannaford, P. (2007) Preferences for self-care or professional advice for minor illness: a discrete choice experiment. *British Journal of General Practice* **57**, 911–917.

Scottish Intercollegiate Guidelines Network (SIGN). (2003) *Diagnosis and management of childhood otitis media in primary care.* http://www.sign.ac.uk/guidelines/fulltext/66/index.html Accessed 10 March 2008.

Silva, P.A., Kirkland, C., Simpson, A., Stewart, J.A. & Williams, S.M. (1982) Some developmental and behavioural problems associated with bilateral otitis media with effusion. *Journal of Learning Disabilities* **15**, 417–421.

A 20-year-old woman with
a sore throat

Emily is the daughter of one of your friends. Your two
families have been on summer holidays together when the
children were younger. She consulted with tonsillitis on
several occasions as a student. You see her in an emergency
appointment in a Friday morning surgery. She has waited
over an hour to see you.

She tells you that she has recently graduated and has
obtained a summer job working in a local insurance call
centre. She and her boyfriend Ben have moved in together,
now that she has a job. Ben is going to the USA for a few
weeks to work in a summer camp. You note from her
record that she last consulted for a prescription for the
contraceptive pill, when she saw one of the other partners.
She tells you she has had a sore throat for 3 days.

What questions do you want to ask Emily?
- Does she feel unwell?
- Does she have a fever or a headache?
- Has she felt nauseated or had any vomiting?
- Is she taking any medications?
- Does she smoke?
- Why has she come about this symptom today?

Emily tells you she feels off colour and is not taking any
medications apart from the pill. She has felt a bit hot at
night, but not had a headache or vomited. She smokes
when she goes to the pub with her friends – only about 5
cigarettes per week.

She asks you to prescribe some antibiotics so that she
does not miss time off work. She will not be paid if she
does not go in and needs the money to clear her student
loan.

Are there any other things you might like to ask?
- What has she treated herself with so far?
- What does she think might be causing it?
- What does she hope you will do for her?

You wonder to yourself whether work is an issue.

She tells you she has taken paracetamol and some over-the-
counter lozenges. These have not worked. She is finding all
the talking at work difficult. She is worried she will not be
able to do her job. She wants a prescription for penicillin:
she knows doctors are reluctant to prescribe antibiotics but
it always worked in the past. She had sore throats a lot as a
teenager. They never got better without antibiotics.

What examination might you want to do and why?
You inspect her throat and check for cervical lymphadenopathy. You are looking for enlarged tonsils with pus in
the crypts (bacterial tonsillitis) or evidence for other
causes of sore throat such as *Candida* (white patches) or
glandular fever, also known as infectious mononucleosis
(palatal haemorrhages).

You should check her temperature and pulse as these
basic measurements will give you an idea of how unwell
Emily is. A high temperature is more likely with a bacterial infection and she may have foetor (bad breath).

When you examine her throat, you find she has red
and enlarged tonsils, but no pus and she has enlarged
cervical nodes. She has no fever or foetor. Her pulse rate
is 68 beats/min.

What are the diagnostic possibilities?
- Viral pharyngitis/tonsillitis
- Bacterial pharyngitis/tonsillitis
- Glandular fever
- Meningitis
- Gonorrhoea
- Pharyngeal thrush

Based on the fact that she is apyrexial without a raised
pulse, you decide she probably has viral tonsillitis.
Although meningitis is not common, it can start with a
sore throat and feeling unwell so this needs to be in the
back of your mind, especially in young adults among
whom the incidence is higher than in older adults.

What do you do now?
Explain your findings to the patient
Your throat is a bit red although there is no sign of bacterial infection.

Explore her understanding of the natural history of the illness
Ninety per cent of sore throats are caused by germs called viruses. Antibiotics do not help viral infections.

Emily says she knows all this and doctors always say the same old stuff, but if she does not get antibiotics it will only get worse and she will end up having more time off work, which she cannot afford to do.

You are in a difficult position here and need to negotiate a management plan.

What options do you have at this point?
• Symptomatic treatment only, such as regular paracetamol and gargling
• Prescribe antibiotics
• Negotiate a delayed prescription

What are the possible consequences of each option?
Symptomatic treatment only
• She may improve
• She may come back and take up another appointment
• She may get worse and develop a complication secondary to a streptococcal infection such as nephritis and blame you for not diagnosing and treating her correctly
• Your continuing relationship may be affected

Prescribe antibiotics
• Her expectation of antibiotics will be increased next time she has a sore throat
• She will be less likely to self-treat minor self-limiting illness
• You will contribute to the development of antibiotic resistance

You decide to give her a delayed or 'back pocket' prescription for antibiotics. This is a prescription a patient can use if the symptoms do not improve within 48 h. The optimum length of treatment is 10 days of penicillin V 250 mg q.i.d. to cover *Streptococcus pyogenes* (or erythromycin 250 mg q.i.d.). These are both long courses of antibiotics to take and four times a day is difficult to remember. Many patients will not complete the course.

Serious complications of tonsillitis (rheumatic fever, nephritis and peritonsillar abscess) are rare and more common in people of low socioeconomic status living in poverty or overcrowded conditions.

What are the other things you should discuss with her at this point?
• Natural history of the condition – her symptoms are likely to resolve in a few days
• 90% are viral
• If she has any allergies to antibiotics
• You discuss the pros and cons of antibiotics (may cause diarrhoea or thrush)
• Antibiotics may shorten the course of the illness slightly
• You explain about the importance of finishing the course of antibiotics if she does take them
• You tell her to use additional contraceptive precautions while taking the antibiotics and for 7 days after

This is also an opportunity to carry out some patient education:
• You discuss smoking cessation – smoking increases the likelihood of upper respiratory tract infections
• You advise her to return if her throat does not settle within 7 days. You may need to consider other diagnoses such as glandular fever then
• If she develops a high fever, vomiting, severe headache or drowsiness she should seek medical help immediately as this might indicate meningitis (Ben needs to know this too)

Emily tells you she will probably get the prescription if her symptoms do not improve very soon. She wonders if she needs her tonsils out? After all she has had this before.

You acknowledge her concern and state that you are willing to discuss the pros and cons of tonsillectomy if it fails to get better.

As she leaves, she hesitantly asks you for a sick note for work.

You discuss the self limiting nature of the illness and advise her that a sick note is not required for the first 7 days of illness. She should be recovered by then. You decide to ask a bit more about work.

Emily says she finds the job boring and wants to spend a bit of time with Ben before he goes to the USA. The company will not accept a self-certificate and she asks you just to write a sick note.

You feel unhappy about this but decide not to compromise your relationship with her. You are tired and she gave you a hard time about the antibiotics.

CASE REVIEW

Sore throat is a very common problem in general practice. Antibiotic resistance is a common problem and the benefits are marginal. Bacterial carriage may be as high as 30%: throat swabs may be misleading (Swartzman 1994). Emily did not have signs of bacterial tonsillitis so antibiotics are not indicated, although they may reduce the duration of symptoms by 24 h.

Although penicillin is cheap, sore throats are common and the number of prescriptions issued is large. Ten per cent of the population are allergic to penicillin.

Complications of tonsillitis such as rheumatic fever are less and less common in the industrialized world. Prescribing might do more harm than good.

The consequences of prescribing are considerable:
- It legitimizes the sore throat as an illness for which you need to see a doctor
- It encourages future attendance for a minor self-limiting condition
- It encourages expectation of a prescription
- It undermines self-management strategies (e.g. gargles, aspirin)

This will impact on doctor workload (Little *et al.* 1997a, b).

Many factors influence whether or not a doctor will prescribe and many of these in primary care are not exclusively clinical. In this case, they might include the doctor's previous relationship with the patient and her family; patient factors such as Emily's wait of 1 h to see the GP and her insistence on antibiotics. Alternatively, the doctor may have had a patient who developed complications as a result of not being given antibiotics, or had a complaint in the past about not prescribing.

Studies have shown that antibiotic prescribing for sore throat by GPs declined between 1995 and 1999 and has remained static since then (Ashworth *et al.* 2004; Smith *et al.* 2004). This has occurred for a number of reasons including patient and doctor education about unnecessary prescribing, increased awareness of the problem of antibiotic resistance and less frequent consultations for sore throat than in the past.

Tonsillectomy may help adults with recurrent tonsillitis (more than five attacks per year) (Little 2007).

KEY POINTS

- Sore throat is a common condition
- Most (90%) sore throats will resolve within 7 days without specific treatment (Del Mar 2000)
- Complications are uncommon
- Antibiotic resistance is rising
- Complications of antibiotic treatment can be significant
- Decisions about treatment have considerable implications for doctors, patients and society
- Patient education is important

References and further reading

Arroll, B., Goodyear-Smith, F., Thomas D.R. & Kerse, N. (2002) Delayed antibiotic prescriptions: what are the experiences and attitudes of physicians and patients? *Journal of Family Practice* 51, 954–959.

Ashworth, M., Latinovic, R., Charlton, J., Cox, K., Rowlands, G. & Gulliford, M. (2004) Why has antibiotic prescribing for respiratory illness declined in primary care? A longitudinal study using the GP Research Database. *Journal of Public Health (Oxford)* **26**, 268–274.

Del Mar, C. (2000) Sore throats and antibiotics. *BMJ* **320**, 130–131.

Graham, A. & Fahey, T. (1999) Sore throat: diagnostic and therapeutic dilemmas. *BMJ* **319**, 173–174.

Little, P. (2007) Recurrent pharyngo-tonsillitis. *BMJ* **334**, 909.

Little, P., Williamson, I., Warner, G., Gould, C., Gantley, M. & Kinmouth, A.L. (1997a) Open randomized trials of prescribing strategies in managing sore throat. *BMJ* **314**, 722–727.

Little, P., Gould, C., Williamson, I., Warner, G., Gantley, M. & Kinmouth, A.L. (1997b) Reattendance and complications in a randomised trial of prescribing strategies for sore throat: the medicalising effect of prescribing antibiotics. *BMJ* **315**, 350–352.

Smith, G.E., Smith, S., Heatlie, H., Bashford, J.N., Hawker, J., Ashcroft, D., *et al.* (2004) What has happened to microbial usage in primary care in the UK since the SMAC report? Description of trends in antimicrobial usage using the GP Research Database. *Journal of Public Health (Oxford)* **26**, 359–364.

Swartzman, P. (1994) Careful prescribing is beneficial. *BMJ* **309**, 1011–1012.

A 35-year-old man with back pain

Ray, a 35-year-old man, attends the surgery one Monday afternoon complaining of back pain. He is a long-distance lorry driver working short haul European routes, for up to a week at a time and he has been troubled with his back in the past.

Ray's family is well known to you. He has three children, the eldest daughter leaving for college in a few months. His wife Ann has rheumatoid arthritis and is disabled. His elderly mother Mavis is also one of your patients. She has osteoarthritis and is housebound.

Ray also has chronic skin problems – labelled dermatitis – from his labouring days. He has always felt the stress of travelling makes his skin problem worse, especially now that he is getting older.

He is a darts champion at the local pub. He slipped on the way home from the pub 5 days ago and tells you his back pain has been worse since.

He drinks about 30 units/week when he is at home at weekends.

What initial questions do you want to ask him?

• How did the pain start (onset)?
• How has it been since (progression)?
• Does anything make it better or worse (relieving and exacerbating factors)?
• What is his past history of low back pain?
• Does he have any other symptoms which may indicate related problems (e.g. skin rash, chronic diarrhoea, ocular problems)?

It is very important to include in your assessment questions that may indicate serious underlying pathology requiring urgent investigation for possible infection, cancer, fracture or spinal cord compression. These features are often termed red flags.

What are the red flags for low back pain?

> **!RED FLAG**
>
> Koes *et al.* (2006); Samanta *et al.* (2003):
> • Onset age under 20 or over 55 years
> • Non-mechanical pain (unrelated to time or activity)
> • Thoracic pain
> • Previous history of carcinoma, steroids, HIV
> • Feeling unwell or presence of other illness
> • Weight loss and fever
> • Neurological symptoms including disturbed gait or saddle anaesthesia
> • Structural spinal deformity (Fig. 3)

Ray tells you that this episode of pain came on gradually over a few weeks. He first noticed it at the end of a long day driving. His back felt stiff and he could hardly get out of the cab. It has been slightly worse since he slipped last weekend, but pretty steady before that.

His back feels best when he is lying down and is worse after long periods of driving or after he has been gardening. He had a little tingling in the left side of his foot at first, but that has now gone and although driving and sitting on the toilet hurts, he has had no other definite symptoms.

Ray tells you he had a previous episode a couple of months ago after lifting a wardrobe when moving his elderly mother into sheltered accommodation.

Does he have any red flags?
No, none of his history indicates serious underlying pathology.

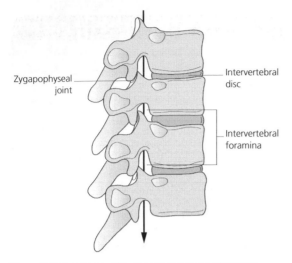

Zygapophyseal joint

Intervertebral disc

Intervertebral foramina

Figure 3 Basic anatomy of lumbar spine and sacroiliac joints.

What features would indicate nerve root problems?

See Box 13. Ray has none of these symptoms at the moment although the tingling in his foot that he experienced initially could have been caused by a nerve root problem.

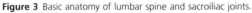

Box 13 **Features indicating nerve root problems**

Koes *et al.* (2006).
- Unilateral leg pain > low back pain
- Pain radiates to foot or toes
- Numbness and paraesthesia in same distribution
- Straight leg raising test induces more leg pain
- Localized neurology (limited to one nerve root)

What other questions might you like to ask Ray?

About his ideas, concerns and expectations:
- Has he any ideas what might be causing his back pain?
- Has he any underlying worries or concerns about it?

Check for features that could indicate risk of chronicity of pain (yellow flags).

What are the yellow flags for low back pain?

!YELLOW FLAG

Yellow flags for occurrence and chronicity of low back pain (Koes *et al.* 2006)

- *Personal factors:* obesity, low level education, high level pain and disability
- *Psychosocial:* distress, depressive mood, somatization
- *Occupational:* job dissatisfaction, requirement of lifting

Ray tells you he finds driving stressful. He was a labourer but it got too heavy for him as he got older, and a mate got him this job as a lorry driver. He is finding it very difficult to sit in the cab all day and he cannot manage to unload the vehicle. He needs to stop to stretch his leg and back when he is driving. This is difficult. He cannot get comfortable in the cab to sleep at night. Some fellow truckers have had the same problem – there is a feeling it is related to the design of the cab.

He worries about Ann when he is away. His daughter goes out a lot. Ray admits he is worried about becoming as disabled as his mother now is. He has been told back problems get worse as you get older. He is worried that he might have a slipped disc. He has heard this can make you immobile.

You decide to examine Ray to help to find out the exact cause of his problem.

General examination: you look at his general appearance and his posture.

He has a beer belly and walks stiffly across the room: he says he has been sitting in the waiting room for 30 min. He has a slight limp with a tilt to the left and is holding the left side of his back. He winces and asks not to sit down as it hurts.

You note a reddish skin rash on the back of his hands. He looks tense and unhappy.

What are the components of a back examination?

See Box 14.

In Ray's case his back appears normal with no muscle wasting, there is no vertebral tenderness. Flexion and extension are reduced, rotation is limited and painful. There is no neurological deficit.

What is the most likely diagnosis?

He is most likely to have benign mechanical back pain. He has no red flag symptoms which would warrant immediate referral and no features indicating nerve root

> **Box 14 Back examination**
>
> - *Look:* posture, mobility, deformity: scoliosis, kyphosis, muscle wasting
> - *Feel:* tenderness over vertebrae
> - *Check movement:* flexion, extension, lateral flexion (finger tip to knee distance), rotation (in sitting position to eliminate flexion at hip), slump test (drop head forward with knee extended, ankle plantar flexed), straight leg raise (heel to bed distance with knee locked in extension, ankle plantar grade)
> - *Check neurology:* perform examination of the motor and sensory dermatomes, including the perineal area

> **Box 15 Treatment plan for back pain**
>
> Adapted from Koes *et al.* (2006).
> - Exploring his ideas, concerns and expectations about cause of disability
> - Reassure him – explain that his back pain is benign and that most improve within 3 months
> - Reassure him that there is no serious pathology and therefore no need for X-ray or blood tests
> - Explain that recurrence is common but unlikely to become a long-term problem
> - Negotiate a treatment plan that involves minimal rest, active mobilization, adequate pain relief and swift return to normal activities
> - Consider analgesics or NSAIDs
> - Explore implications for family and work and address these issues if appropriate

pathology. He might have osteoarthritic change in the lumbar spine which has given rise to brief symptoms of disc prolapse with nerve root irritation.

Does this condition warrant any further investigation?

Blood tests and imaging are not indicated as they will not help with the diagnosis or management plan.

You explain to Ray that you think that he has mechanical low back pain and that this does not require any further investigation. He is not very happy with this as he wants to know what has caused it.

You think that the stress his lifestyle places on his family and wife is one of the keys to helping Ray to cope. You know that he does not enjoy being away from home and he worries about how his wife and mother cope on their own. You know that his daughter is feeling under pressure and is looking forward to leaving home for college.

How do you decide on an appropriate treatment plan?

The plan should be evidence based. Koes *et al.* (2006) summarize the treatments that are known to be beneficial versus those that are not. Treatments known to be beneficial in acute back pain are staying active and non-steroidal anti-inflammatory drugs (NSAIDs). In chronic back pain, exercise therapy and intensive multidisciplinary treatment programmes are of benefit.

Utilization of appropriate guidelines is important although there can be many to choose from – at present there are more than 11 national guidelines for acute low back pain (Koes *et al.* 2006).

What is an appropriate treatment plan for Ray's back pain?

See Box 15.

> *After further discussion he decides to have a week off work and asks for a sick note. He also says that he needs some painkillers as he does not feel paracetamol is strong enough.*

What factors might influence your choice of painkillers?

- Age
- Other medications
- Other medical conditions
- Possible side-effects and interactions

His past medical history might mean that he is unable to take anti-inflammatory medication such as ibuprofen because of asthma or an ulcer.

> *He asks for codeine.*

What should you tell him about codeine?

You should tell him this may make him sleepy and that he should consider whether it might have an effect on his driving. You suggest he takes it only in the week he is off work and does not mix it with alcohol. You should also warn him that he may become constipated and so to make sure that his intake of fibre is high.

What other things might you like to discuss?

You might mention lifting and handling, adjustment of driving seat and, as longer term issues, weight loss, exercise, alcohol reduction and carer support.

> *Outcome. Four weeks later he returns. His back is worse. His daughter has just left home and his wife needs him to care for her. He does not feel ready to go back to work.*

He gets in touch with the union and they say he may have a case for work-related injury. The case takes 18 months during which time he is told to stay off sick. He does not attend for a physiotherapy appointment and continues to request analgesia in the form of codeine.

He never returns to work. He starts to claim benefit for disability. Social Services care for him and his wife. His mother has a fall and dies soon after. His daughter never returns from college, but gets a job in London. From time to time you see him coming home from the pub in the late afternoon.

CASE REVIEW

Back pain is an extremely common problem in primary care. NICE (2007) reports that a survey in 1998 showed that 40% of all adults had experienced low back pain lasting longer than 1 day in the previous 12 months. Back pain has a major cost implication as it costs the NHS more than £1000 million/year and it has a major cost to industry in terms of days lost at work, with lost production costing in excess of £3500 million/year (NICE 2007).

The prognosis is usually good. Ninety per cent of cases will have resolved in 3 months; recurrences are common, only 5% go on to become chronic (Koes *et al.* 2006).

Medicalization is often the worst thing to do. Interventions and therapies aim to manage disability, help people to cope with everyday life including remaining at work, reduce distress and minimize recurrence (NICE 2007). If the patient has red flags, referral is indicated urgently. The clinical guidance for imaging is to restrict it to cases with red flag conditions or suspected nerve root pathology (Royal College of Radiologists 2007).

Cauda equina syndrome is a low back pain emergency. It presents with a history of saddle anaesthesia, recent onset of bladder or bowel dysfunction, recent onset of faecal incontinence. Examination findings include severe or progressive neurological deficit in lower extremities, unexpected laxity of anal sphincter, perineal and/or peri-anal sensory loss, major motor weakness. If one or more of these are present, the patient should be referred immediately.

Refer for specialist assessment other back problems where:
- Serious spinal pathology is suspected
- There is progressive neurological deficit
- There is nerve root pain not resolving after 6 weeks
- Underlying inflammatory disease such as ankylosing spondylitis is suspected
- Simple back pain but has not resumed normal activities in 3 months

Ray demonstrates that giving a sick note for a self-limiting condition has implications. Social, psychological and occupational factors contribute to the outcome and should be assessed using the yellow flag system. Ray's fears of disability, his responsibility for his wife and his beliefs about how the back pain was caused (work) have had effects on his recovery. Long-term sickness and disability are often associated with undiagnosed depression. His continuing use of alcohol and analgesics may reflect this.

KEY POINTS

- Back pain is an extremely common problem in primary care
- Prognosis is usually good. Ninety per cent of cases will have resolved in 3 months
- Patients should be assessed to check for red flags that could indicate serious underlying pathology and yellow flags that would suggest features leading to chronicity
- Do not medicalize unless there is clear evidence of a serious problem
- It is vital to involve the patient in the management plan

References

Koes, B.W., van Tulder, M.W. & Thomas, S. (2006) Diagnosis and treatment of low back pain. *BMJ* **332**, 1430–1434.

National Institute for Health and Clinical Excellence (NICE). (2007) http://www.nice.org.uk/nicemedia/pdf/LowBackPain_FinalScope.pdf Accessed on 28 November 2007.

The Royal College Radiologists. (2007) *Making the best use of clinical radiology services; referral guidelines.* The Royal College of Radiologists: London.

Samanta, J., Kendall, J. & Samanta, S. (2003) Chronic low back pain. *BMJ* **326**, 535.

A 62-year-old woman with a painful shoulder

Rosemary is a 62-year-old retired civil servant who comes to see you in the surgery looking tired and uncomfortable. She tells you that she has pain and stiffness in her left shoulder. She thinks this started when her elderly Labrador dog pulled suddenly on the lead a few months ago but she cannot be sure. On reflection she had had a bit of aching prior to that.

She has come as the pain is getting worse and is keeping her awake at night. Worse than that, she is finding it difficult to put on her bra and cardigan, and cannot put her hair up easily. She is finding it difficult to open the car door.

You know that she is fiercely independent and extremely stoical. She lives alone. She had breast cancer 4 years ago and made a swift recovery, impressing everyone with her determination to resume normal life as soon as possible.

What are the initial questions that you would like to ask Rosemary?

See Box 16.

She tells you that she feels well though tired from lack of sleep. She is right-handed, but uses her left arm more as she had stiffness in her right shoulder after her mastectomy.

Box 16 History of shoulder pain

After Mitchell *et al.* (2005).
- Onset and characteristic of pain?
- Is the pain at rest or on movement, or both?
- Is there pain at night?
- Any neck, thoracic or other upper limb pain?
- Are you right or left handed?
- Is there any history of trauma, or joint instability (dislocation)?
- Occupation and sporting activities?
- How do you feel in yourself? Any fever, weight loss, rash or respiratory symptoms?
- Any significant comorbidity? Drug treatments?
- Any problems with this shoulder in the past?
- Any problems with any other joints?

She still has a little lymphoedema in that arm. A hospital check up 3 months ago was clear. You notice she has a past history of type 2 diabetes.

What is your differential diagnosis of shoulder pain?

Mitchell *et al.* (2005).
- Glenohumeral problem (osteoarthritis shoulder, capsulitis, frozen shoulder)
- Rotator cuff disorder
- Referred pain from neck
- Metastatic problem
- Acromioclavicular joint disease
- Polymyalgia rheumatica
- Infection
- Referred cardiac ischaemia, referred diaphragmatic pain
- Primary malignancy – apical lung cancer

Does Rosemary have any indicators of serious underlying pathology?

Yes, she has a past history of breast cancer.

!RED FLAG

Indicators of serious underlying pathology (Mitchell *et al.* 2005):
- History of cancer; symptoms and signs of cancer; unexplained deformity, mass or swelling? Tumour
- Red skin, fever, systemically unwell? Infection
- Trauma, epileptic fit, electric shock; loss of rotation and normal shape? Unreduced dislocation
- Trauma, acute disabling pain and significant weakness, positive drop arm test? Acute rotator cuff tear
- Unexplained significant sensory or motor deficit? Neurological lesion

What examination should you perform?

See Box 17.

> ### Box 17 Examination of the shoulder joint
>
> After Mitchell *et al.* (2005).
> - Examine neck, axilla and chest wall
> - Assess range of movement of cervical spine
> - Inspect shoulders for swelling, wasting and deformity
> - Palpate sternoclavicular, acromioclavicular and glenohumeral joints for tenderness, swelling, warmth and crepitus
> - Compare power, stability, range of movement (active and passive) of both shoulders
> - Look for painful arc (70–120° active abduction)
> - Test passive external rotation
> - Drop arm test – patient lowers abducted arm slowly to waist

She looks well and has a normal range of neck movements. On examination of her axilla and chest wall she has a mastectomy scar; no other abnormalities are found.

Her shoulder is not swollen and there is no muscle wasting. She has some non-specific tenderness on palpation of the glenohumeral joint but it is not hot. There is crepitus also present. You find that Rosemary has greatly reduced movement generally, particularly in forward flexion and external rotation. See Fig. 4.

What investigations could you perform?

- Full blood count, plasma viscosity to rule out polymyalgia

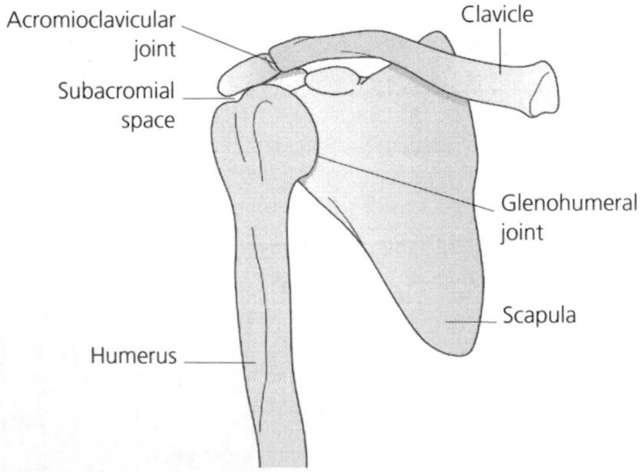

- Shoulder X-ray for persistent shoulder pain unresponsive to conservative treatment (Royal College of Radiologists 2007)

| *She has a normal plasma viscosity and shoulder X-ray.*

What is your diagnosis?

Left frozen shoulder or adhesive capsulitis is likely as it presents with a precedent history of non-adhesive capsulitis, deep joint pain and restricted activities caused by impaired external rotation. The typical age range of presentation is 40–65 years (Mitchell *et al.* 2005).

How should you manage her?

- Explain the anatomy, natural history and causation. It is common in her age group and is where the tissues tighten around the joint preventing movement. It usually ends in resolution. It could be followed up with an information leaflet from the Arthritis Research Campaign (www.arc.org).
- Explore her ideas, concerns and expectations of treatment and recovery. There are three phases (Box 18) and it may take up to 2 years to resolve fully, although sometimes symptoms persist for longer (Mitchell *et al.* 2005).
- Negotiate a plan of action. Encourage mobilization and self-help, explain that there is no evidence that physiotherapy alone is of benefit but with corticosteroid intra-articular injection there may be short-term benefit.
- Ask about social history. She may need help at home.
- Safety net. Arrange for follow-up to ensure symptoms are settling and no additional problems are emerging.

Figure 4 The shoulder complex of joints.

> ### Box 18 Three phases of clinical presentation of frozen shoulder
>
> Dias *et al.* (2005).
> 1 *Painful freezing phase:* pain and stiffness around the shoulder, nagging constant pain worse at night, little response to non-steroidal anti-inflammatory drugs (NSAIDs)
> 2 *Adhesive phase:* pain gradually subsides, stiffness remains, pain at extremes of movement, no external rotation
> 3 *Resolution phase:* spontaneous improvement of range of movement

Outcome. Rosemary becomes quite low as a result of the pain in her shoulder. You see her fairly regularly for analgesia and support. Physiotherapy and injection do not help. She loses weight and energy. A friend has to drive her to appointments and look after her dog. She is no longer able to go to bridge evenings. She loses confidence.

The following year she asks for a home visit. You notice she is moving her arm more freely but she wants you to check her dry cough and when you examine her chest you notice she has a small nodule at the lower part of her mastectomy scar. She copes well with her diagnosis of metastatic breast cancer and when you see her for a medication review she is fairly well and on her way to a card party. Her arm movement is normal.

CASE REVIEW

The diagnosis of shoulder problems is complex and often several conditions coexist (Mitchell *et al.* 2005).

Frozen shoulder is common and usually self-limiting. There are three hallmarks of frozen shoulder: shoulder stiffness, severe pain even at night and near-complete loss of passive and active external rotation. History and examination are the keys to diagnosis. In this case, frozen shoulder was likely because of the history of minimal trauma, surgery to that arm, her family history of diabetes and the classic findings of restriction of flexion and external rotation. Usually, all laboratory tests are normal (Dias *et al.* 2005), as was the case here.

Physiotherapy with injection might help but the key to treatment is helping her to cope with the problem until it resolves spontaneously. Refactory cases should be referred for manipulation under anaesthesia or arthroscopic release (Dias *et al.* 2005).

KEY POINTS

- Adhesive capsulitis presents as shoulder stiffness, severe pain even at night and near-complete loss of passive and active external rotation
- Typical age range of presentation is 40–65 years
- All laboratory tests are normal
- Key to treatment is helping patient cope with the problem until it resolves spontaneously
- Physiotherapy with intra-articular injection may provide some short-term benefit

References

Dias, R., Cutts, C. & Massoud, S. (2005) Clinical review: frozen shoulder. *BMJ* **331**, 1453–1456.

Mitchell, C., Abajo, A., Hay, E. & Carr, A. (2005) Shoulder pain: diagnosis and management in primary care. *BMJ* **331**, 1124–1128.

The Royal College of Radiologists. (2007) *Making the best use of clinical radiology services: referral guidelines.* The Royal College of Radiologists: London.

www.arc.org.uk/about-arth/booklets/60396039.atm

Case 10 A 35-year-old woman with knee pain

Nazreen arrived from Pakistan 5 years ago. She is married with no children. She is a quiet young woman who works as a tailoress in her husband's clothing business. She has consulted intermittently with joint pains over the past few years.

She tells you that she has pain in her right knee. The left knee feels fine. This is causing problems at work, as it is aching and she is not able to complete her work sometimes. Her knee aches when she is sitting and also when climbing stairs. She cannot manage the house properly. This is causing tension at home.

What questions might you want to ask Nazreen?
- Has there been any history of trauma?
- Is the knee hot or red?
- Is it swollen?
- Does it ever lock, click or give way?
- Is it painful all the time?
- Are any other joints affected?
- How does she feel in herself?
- Is there any family history of joint problems?
- What are her concerns about the knee?
- Has it happened before?

She denies any recent injury or trauma, and she tells you that she thinks it swells occasionally but is never hot or red. She feels that it does give way although she has never fallen. She does not feel a click and nor does it lock. She reiterates that is hurts after standing at work, sitting with a bent knee for long periods and going up and down the stairs. She says she feels well in herself. Nazreen is worried that she will end up having problems walking as her mother has joint pains and is quite disabled with 'arthritis'.

What is your differential diagnosis?
- Anterior knee pain
- Mechanical knee pain
- Osteoarthritis
- Inflammatory arthritis
- Physical presentation of a psychosocial problem

What examination should you do?
General examination
You watch her walk from the waiting room.

She looks well and is wearing a black shalwar kameez. She walks normally, with a normal gait and no deformity. She appears overweight and has a body mass index (BMI) of 29. She is apyrexial.

Knee examination
See Boxes 19 and 20; Fig. 5.

Box 19 McMurrays test

Adapted from http://www.fpnotebook.com/ORT102.htm

Starting position
- Ask the patient to lie supine
- Flex the knee to 45 degrees
- Flex the hip to 45 degrees
- Hold the lower leg securely
- One hand on the ankle and one hand on the knee

Medial meniscal assessment
Assess for pain on palpation
Palpate the medial joint line with the knee flexed
Assess for a 'click' suggestion meniscus relocation;
    Apply valgus stress to the flexed knee
    Externally rotate the leg (toes pointing outwards)
    Extend the knee whilst still in valgus

Lateral meniscal assessment
Repeat the above with varus stress and internally rotate the knee

---

You perform the knee examination on both sides, comparing the normal with the affected side. You remember that referred pain from the hip is a cause of knee pain, you also check hip movement.

PART 2: CASES

> Box 20 Knee examination

Inspection
- *Standing:* check for swelling, redness, deformity, muscle wasting
- *Supine:* check for the same including effusion, patellar position and normal bony contours

Palpation
- Check for heat
- Effusions including the patellar tap
- Joint line tenderness for meniscal injuries

Movement
- Check for range of movement of flexion, extension and hyperextension
- Check for passive active and active resisted movements

Ligaments
- Check collateral in flexion and 20° extension
- Check cruciate ligaments with anterior and posterior draw tests, Lachman test (Fig. 5) and pivot test

Menisci
- Check for joint line tenderness and perform McMurray's test

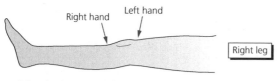

Left hand stabilizes distal femur, right hand holds proximal tibia

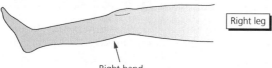

Right hand pulls tibia forwards, positive test if there is movement, with a 'soft' end point

Figure 5 Lachman's test.

Examination of the knees reveals minor valgus deformity and no asymmetry of the knees. Palpation reveals no swelling or effusion and no joint line tenderness. She has a full range of movement, both active and passive. There is no crepitus. There is also no ligament instability demonstrable as the Lachman's test is negative. The McMurray's test is also normal with no pain or clicking over the joint line which

would suggest a meniscal problem. However, the anterior knee pain is reproduced when you ask her to go up and down the step to the examination couch.

What is your working diagnosis now?
- Mechanical knee pain
- Anterior knee pain

You check for psychosocial problems and work stresses. What questions might you ask to do this?
- How exactly is it affecting her life?
- Are there any things she avoids doing?
- What does her job involve?
- Does she have any other hobbies?
- Does she have any other worries?
- Does she ever feel low or unhappy?

She admits she is not very happy. She feels homesick and has not had a baby as quickly as she would like. Sometimes her husband loses his temper with her. Her mother-in-law still expects her to help at home even if her knee hurts. Her mother has joint pains and has been told she has arthritis.

What is your plan for management?
Exclude Red flags

> **!RED FLAG**
> - Haemarthrosis
> - Instability
> - Fever

Your examination has not shown any of these features.

Assess Yellow flags

> **!YELLOW FLAG**
> - Occupational history
> - Effect on job
> - Effect at home
> - Degree of pain

Nazreen has already told you that standing at work makes the pain worse and she is having trouble completing her work on occasion. She says the pain is 'aching' in nature and on a scale of 1–10 (with 10 being the most severe) it is about 5.

You ask her if she has tried any painkillers?

Nazreen says she has tried rubbing in Deep Heat cream which a friend gave her which has helped a little. She has not taken any tablets at all.

You consider whether this may be a presentation of psychological distress as depression is a common problem in primary care and Nazreen has already admitted to you that she is stressed and anxious about not getting pregnant. You ask some screening questions (Box 21) and arrange to review her. She is worried about the possibility of not being able to walk.

Box 21 Questions used to screen for depression

- During the last month have you been feeling down, depressed and hopeless?
- During the last month have you been bothered by having little interest or pleasure in doing things?

What is your diagnosis?

You decide anterior knee pain resulting from patello-femoral maltracking is the most likely diagnosis. This is caused by the presence of a minor valgus deformity suggesting that the patellar does not move smoothly through the femoral groove. The fact that the pain is reproduced when going up and down stairs, after prolonged sitting and there is no other significant pathology further supports this diagnosis.

What are you going to say to Nazreen?

You explain that you have not found any major problem with the knee but she may have kneecaps that are a little unstable. You would like to refer her to see a physiotherapist for some exercise to strengthen the muscles which support the knee. This should help with the problem but you think she should try and lose weight as well to reduce the strain on the knees. You suggest she takes paracetamol if the pain is severe.

Nazreen is relieved it is not a serious joint problem. She says she will try and lose weight but this is difficult for her as she does all the cooking and both she and her husband eat a large meal in the evening. She has not tried taking any exercise because of her painful knee.

What is your management plan?

You decide to arrange a physiotherapy assessment to assess postural problems, improve vastus medialis muscle strengthening and advise Nazreen to book an appointment with the practice nurse for weight loss advice. You tell her that you will arrange for some blood tests and will let her know if any of the results come back as abnormal.

Outcome. The blood test results are all normal and do not show any sign of gout or infection. The plasma viscosity level is normal which rules out an infective or inflammatory process. You ask her to make an appointment in a few weeks to see you after she has had the physiotherapy.

CASE REVIEW

Anterior knee pain is the most likely diagnosis. This is usually caused by abnormal biomechanical forces through the patellar complex, and is very common. Her history of intermittent pain, worse after sitting or going up stairs, is characteristic.

Meniscal or anterior cruciate injury is unlikely because of the absence of trauma. These are usually caused by high impact sports and often there is a clear history of a 'pop' or a 'crack', described as the noise made when opening a can of coke.

The lack of warmth or swelling makes infection unlikely and the normal blood tests confirm this. However, in view of her history of having lived in Pakistan, it is important to be sure tuberculosis is considered.

Hip problems can present with knee pain but is unlikely in Nazreen's case as she has a normal painless gait. Osteoarthritis would be very unlikely in someone this age without a history of trauma.

It is important to check her ideas concerns and expectations; she may have worries about her mobility (because of her mother) or there may be some other underlying problem, such as depression. She has given some hints in terms of impaired fertility and marital tension.

This seems to be a cry for help. As a GP, it is important to be on the look out for this. Nazreen went on to be a victim of domestic violence.

Four months later Nazreen attends with widespread bruising. She tells you she is the victim of domestic violence. She has joint pains all over. She is feeling suicidal.

You record her injuries in the notes, arrange a crisis mental health assessment and placement at a women's refuge.

Reference

McMurray's technique. http://www.fpnotebook.com/ORT102.htm Accessed on 4 December 2007.

KEY POINTS

- Knee pain is very common in primary care
- Most knee problems are diagnosed on the history
- Refer hot or swollen knees after trauma as this may indicate infection or bleeding, both of which require urgent treatment
- Other knee problems can generally be managed in practice
- Remember knee pain as a presentation for a hip problem
- Biomechanical assessment is often helpful
- Joint pain may be the presenting symptom for other problems and a full psychosocial assessment is a good idea
- In cases of physical abuse or assault, accurate record keeping is essential

Case 11 A 78-year-old male with rash on trunk

Bill Stevenson rarely attends the GP. He comes to see you with some chest pain that he says it is coming from the surface of his chest and it started after he had been digging his vegetable patch. He does not like taking painkillers and so has only taken a few paracetamol but it is keeping him awake at night. He finds the character of his pain difficult to describe but says that it feels like he has burnt himself and it is there constantly. On examination there is nil of note.

Are there further questions that you would like to ask?

- Is this the first time that he has had pain like this?
- Is it on one side of his chest or both?
- Does the pain go anywhere else?
- Does anything make it worse or better?
- Has he been short of breath or had any palpitations?
- Has he had any other symptoms with it?
- Has he felt unwell?

He says that the pain is a new experience to him as he is normally fit and well. He supposes that he was just overdoing it in the garden and so he has 'pulled something'. It is only on the right side and does not travel anywhere else. Nothing makes it better, not even the paracetamol, and it is there the whole time. He has not been short of breath or had any palpitations but he has been feeling generally 'out of sorts'.

What is the differential diagnosis?

- *Cardiac or respiratory pathology:* this is unlikely as it is constant and there is no shortness of breath or palpitations
- *Gastrointestinal pathology:* burning pain is sometimes used to describe oesophagitis or gastritis but Mr Stevenson says that it feels like it is coming from the surface of his chest
- *Musculoskeletal pathology:* it could be a muscular sprain from digging but it is a burning pain and also the examination does not fit with this
- *Shingles:* a possible diagnosis but there are no skin changes and so no objective evidence of infection although the pain could be an acute neuritis prodrome to shingles
- *Malignancy:* this is very unlikely given the short duration

Further questioning confirms that there are no associated cardiac, respiratory or gastrointestinal symptoms. He has not lost any weight and felt well until the pain started.

Which are the most likely diagnoses and what would be your course of action?

Acute neuritis is the most likely diagnosis although some components fit with a chest wall sprain. To help with the pain you could give him a stronger analgesic (e.g. co-codamol) and suggest a review appointment if he develops a rash, the symptoms do not settle or if he has further concern.

He returns 1 week later. He did not take the co-codamol for long as it made him constipated and repeats that he does not like taking tablets. He has come back as he has developed a red patch on his chest but he thinks this may be from the Deep Heat or the hot water bottles that he has been using to help with the pain.

What are the characteristics of the rash that would confirm a diagnosis of shingles (herpes zoster)?

A shingles rash looks red and has vesicles containing clear fluid along the distribution of a dermatome (Fig. 6; Plate 2, facing p. 56).

You examine him and there is a red rash with crops of vesicles. It lies on the right-hand side of his chest in a well-defined patch.

What advice should you give to him?

You should advise him of the diagnosis and ask him to start taking pain relief as needed. Ice packs may help reduce the pain rather than heat.

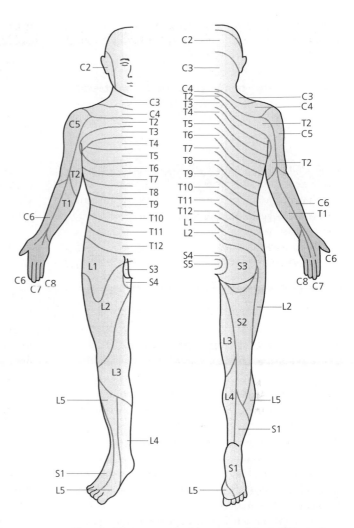

Figure 6 Approximate distribution of the dermatomes on the anterior and posterior aspects of the body.

PART 2: CASES

You should offer him some simple laxatives to counteract the constipation.

Advise him that it is infectious but only if others have contact with the vesicle fluid. Particular at-risk groups are the immunosuppressed, children who have not had chickenpox and pregnant women.

Finally, ask him to return if the rash does not heal within a month or the pain does not subside.

A patient advice leaflet could be obtained from www.patient.co.uk.

Should he be prescribed an antiviral and if so which one?

Antivirals should be started within 72 h of onset of rash and be given in a course of 7–10 days. Aciclovir is effective and a meta-analysis showed that 800 mg five times daily reduced the duration of pain, particularly in the elderly (Wood *et al.* 1996).

You decide to prescribe him oral aciclovir 800 mg five times daily for 1 week (Box 22; *BNF* 2006).

> **Box 22 Effects of systemic antiviral therapy on shingles**
>
> *BNF* (2006).
> - Reduce the severity and duration of pain
> - Reduce complications
> - Reduce viral shedding

What are the side-effects of aciclovir to warn him about?

Nausea, vomiting, abdominal pain, diarrhoea, headache, fatigue, rash, urticaria, pruritus and photosensitivity are the most common side-effects.

After hearing about how often he will have to take the medication and about the possible side-effects that could occur he says that he would rather just chance his luck.

What are the other reasons for patients not taking their medication?

See Box 23.

> ### Box 23 Reasons for poor patient concordance
>
> Corlett (1996).
> * Not knowing how to take the medication
> * Not understanding the importance of the medication
> * Taking several medications
> * Worries about anticipated or experienced side-effects
> * Forgetting
> * Impaired physical function

How could you help with patient concordance in this case?

You could openly discuss with him that he does not like taking tablets and that you know that you are asking him to take something several times a day but it will only be for 1 week.

You should state the reasons for the medication saying that it will make him less infectious and that it is likely to reduce the severity and duration of the pain. It will also reduce complications including scarring, secondary infection and ulceration.

You could also tell him that you would not prescribe him any medication unless you thought that it would be beneficial to him.

Finally, you could give him a patient information leaflet about shingles.

Bill reluctantly agrees to the treatment and takes the prescription. He returns 3 weeks later. The rash has healed but he is still in pain despite the co-codamol which is still making him constipated. The other drugs made him feel a bit sick but he 'stuck with it' because you told him that it was important to complete the course. He is a bit angry as you said that it should stop the pain but it hurts even when his shirt brushes against his skin and he has been forced to wear a shirt in bed to stop the covers rubbing.

What is the likely diagnosis?

He is likely to have developed postherpetic neuralgia.

What is the character of neuropathic pain?

See Box 24.

> ### Box 24 Neuropathic pain is often described as
>
> Higson (2005).
> * Shooting
> * Stabbing
> * Electric
> * Searing
> * Worse at night

What examination should you perform?

Examination of the peripheral nervous system is indicated and may demonstrate paraesthesia along with dysthetic pain. Paraesthesiae are abnormal sensory changes that are not painful and dysthetic pains are unpleasant sensations that are painful. A full examination would include a cotton swab to test light touch, a tuning fork to test vibration sense and a metal roller for pressure (Higson 2005).

On examination, light touch induces pain over the dermatome where the rash was, you decide that testing for vibration or pressure will not further your diagnosis or management plan, will only induce more discomfort and so do not perform this part of the examination.

What treatment should you give him?

The most appropriate method of reducing pain from postherpetic neuralgia is by the use of antiviral agents (Cope & Kudesia 2005). These have already been given and as simple analgesics have not been effective you decide to try him on amitriptyline. This should be given initially in a small night-time dose of 25 mg and gradually increased this to 75 mg nocte. It should be remembered that it can cause many side-effects including difficulty with urinating that could be a particular problem if the patient has prostatic symptoms (*BNF* 2006).

Occasionally, strong opioids are required (Allen 2006). Patients with severe pain should be referred for specialist pain management.

What should you explain to him about this medication?

You should explain that it is from a class of drugs that is often used to treat depression but that it also can reduce

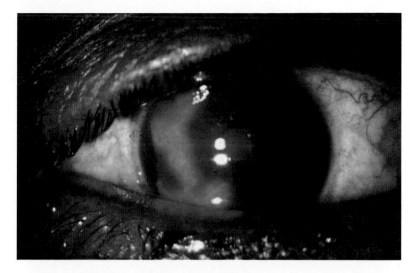

Plate 1 The eye. From www.opt.indiana.
edu/ce/hsk/index.htm Reproduced with
kind permission from Dr Brad Sutton,
Indianapolis Eye Care Center, USA
(p. 31).

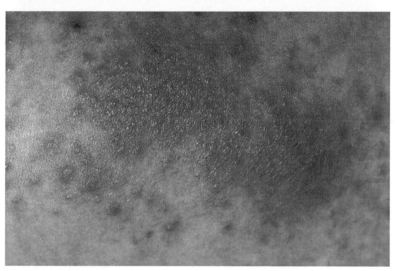

Plate 2 Herpes zoster (p. 54).

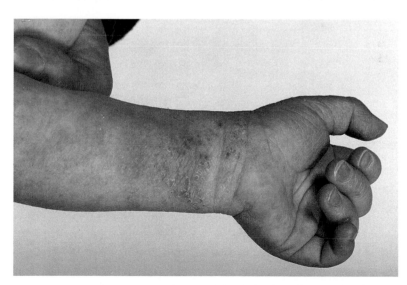

Plate 3 Eczema (p. 59). From du Vivier,
A. (2002) *Dermatology: Pocket Picture
Book*. Blackwell Science, with permission.

Facing p. 56.

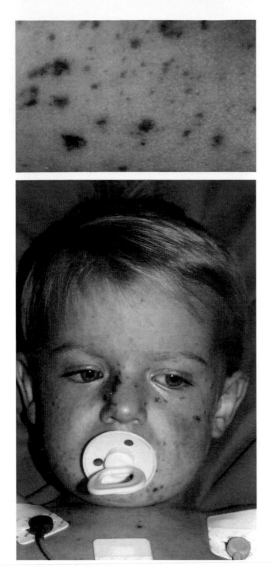

Plate 4 Meningococcal rash (p. 63). From Newell, S.J. & Darling, J.C. (2008) *Lecture Notes in Paediatrics*, 8th edn. Blackwell Publishing, with permission.

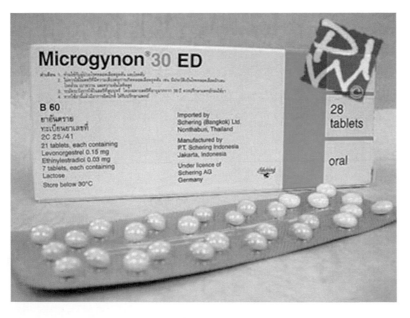

Plate 5 Contraceptive pill Microgynon-30 ED (p. 162). Image from http://beauty.the-nagasaki.com/images/MGYNED.jpg Accessed on 26 November 2007.

pain by acting on the pathway that takes the pain signals to the brain. You should also explain that unfortunately he may experience some side-effects and so you are starting him on a small dose to minimize these. You should carefully describe the side-effects by referring to the *BNF* or you could print off a patient information leaflet from www.patient.co.uk.

Outcome. He calls the surgery to tell you that the amitriptyline is settling his pain but complains of a dry mouth and feeling dopey when he gets up in the night to urinate. He is prepared to put up with the side-effects as the pain is easing. After several weeks he is able to stop the amitriptyline with no return of his discomfort.

CASE REVIEW

The varicella-zoster virus causes the primary infection chickenpox. The initial infection generates immunoglobulin G (IgG) which is protective against further chickenpox but the virus can establish life-long latency in neural tissue. Reactivation causes a painful localized cutaneous eruption; this is known as shingles. This most often occurs in those over 50 years old. If it is recurrent or occurs in someone young it should cause suspicion of poor T-cell immunity.

It should be remembered that if the trigeminal nerve is affected ophthalmic zoster can be complicated by keratitis or iritis and so should be referred for specialist treatment (Higson 2005).

Mr Stevenson was very unfortunate as he developed pain both before and after the rash. Pain most commonly occurs as a prodrome but may also occur for weeks or months after the infection. The prodrome is called acute neuritis and if it occurs for more than 4 weeks after the lesions it is called postherpetic neuralgia (Higson 2005).

Neuropathic pain is caused by a pathological process causing nerve injury and it follows the nerve distribution. Pain is caused by infection of the nerve root that is situated close to the spinal cord but the pain will be perceived peripherally. The symptoms lead to loss of function and autonomic changes may occur e.g. sweating (Higson 2005).

Mr Stevenson does not like taking medication and several different drug treatments had to be negotiated with him to manage this illness. There are many ways of helping with patient concordance including:

- Exploring patient views on the possibility of having to take medication
- Informing patients of the pros and cons of taking and not taking medication
- Involving the patient in the treatment decision-making process (Elwyn *et al.* 2003).

If Mr Stevenson's condition had not improved he could have been offered support and information from the Neuropathy Trust (www.neuropathy-trust.org). Many illnesses and conditions have patient support groups and these can prove to be very useful as they give patients independent sources of help and advice.

KEY POINTS

- Herpes zoster rash is usually unilateral, affects any dermatome, lasts 2–4 weeks
- Patients should be advised to avoid contact with the immunosuppressed (e.g. those on steroids or receiving chemotherapy), children who have not had chickenpox or pregnant women in case they pass on the infection
- Systemic antivirals should be prescribed within 72 h of rash onset to reduce pain, complication and viral shedding
- Pain as a prodrome is called acute neuritis and if it occurs for more than 4 weeks after the lesions it is called postherpetic neuralgia
- Pain may be helped by anti-inflammatories or simple compound analgesics but often tricyclic antidepressants or anti-epileptic medications are required

References

Allen, S. (2006) *Neuropathic pain. GP Pocket Guide.* Medical Imprint, London.

British National Formulary, 52nd edn. (2006) Royal Pharmaceutical Society of Great Britain. RPS Publishing and BMJ Publishing Group, London.

Cope, A. & Kudesia, G. (2005) Recommended management of herpetic skin infections. *Prescriber* **16**, 31–41.

Corlett, A.J. (1996) Caring for older people: aids to compliance with medication. *BMJ* **313**, 926–929.

Elwyn, G., Edwards, A. & Britten, N. (2003) 'Doing prescribing': how doctors can be more effective. *BMJ* **327**, 864–867.

Higson, N. (2005) Neuropathic pain: should we be taking a fresh look? *The New Generalist* **3**, 21–24.

Wood, M.J., Kay, R., Dworkin, R.H., Soong, S.J. & Whitley, R.J. (1996) Oral aciclovir therapy accelerates pain resolution in patient with herpes zoster: a meta-analysis of placebo-controlled trials. *Clinical Infectious Diseases* **22**, 341–347.

Case 12 — A 2-year-old boy with a rash

Mrs Begum comes to see you bringing with her Mohammed, her 2-year-old son, who has had bad eczema since he was a baby. You have seen Mrs Begum on numerous occasions as two of her other five children have quite severe asthma. You last saw Mohammed to prescribe emollients for his skin a couple of months ago.

At the moment Mohammed is going through a bad phase and constantly scratching at his skin. Mrs Begum tells you tearfully that she is up several times in the night because Mohammed is crying and his skin is hot and inflamed and sometimes bleeding. Mrs Begum looks exhausted and Mohammed is fretful and flushed.

What do you need to ask Mrs Begum before you examine Mohammed?
- How long has Mohammed's skin been worse?
- Are there any precipitating factors (triggers) she has noticed that make his skin flare up?
- Has he been unwell recently?
- Is he allergic to anything?
- What does she usually use to moisturize his skin?

Mohammed has had a slight cold in the last week, with a fever in the afternoons and evenings. Mrs Begum has not noticed any particular things that make his skin worse although she does think it is always bad when he is unwell with a temperature. She usually uses aqueous cream for his skin and Oilatum Plus in the bath but does not find these very effective currently. She is not sure if he is allergic to anything.

What examination do you need to carry out?
- Mohammed's general appearance and temperature
- The pattern of the eczema – is it confined to the flexures (antecubital and popliteal fossae and often in the neck) or more widespread?

- Take his temperature, examine his chest and check his ears as he has had a recent cold

Mohammed is very uncooperative which makes examining him very difficult. He cries as soon as you approach him and appears frightened and miserable. What can you do to make him more comfortable while you have a look at him?

Make sure he is sitting on his mother's lap where he feels safe and give him a toy to hold or a baby book to look at and talk in a soothing tone. You can also ask Mrs Begum to try and distract him while you carry out the examination.

Mohammed is an overweight toddler and feverish with a temperature of 37.5°C. He has very dry skin with widespread eczema on his neck, the back of both pinnae, his wrists and the extensor aspects of his forearms and legs. In places that he can reach to scratch his skin is excoriated with crusting and signs of bleeding, particularly on his legs and arms (Plate 3, facing p. 56). His chest is clear and ear drums appear red (he screams while you are trying to examine him) but he has no other signs of ear infection.

What are you going to do next?
It is extremely distressing and exhausting having a fractious toddler with eczema and Mohammed is in the vicious cycle of itch–scratch–itch. The fact he is overweight will exacerbate the problem as he is likely to sweat more and get hot at night, which will also make his skin worse.

Eczema that has crusting is almost certainly infected so he will need an oral antibiotic such as flucloxacillin 125 mg q.i.d. for 10–14 days to treat this. Flucloxacillin is effective because it treats *Staphylococcus aureus*, a common cause of skin infections.

He should also have paracetamol 120 mg to bring his temperature down.

Could this be eczema herpeticum?

Occasionally, eczema becomes secondarily infected with herpes simplex. In this case, there are no crusted vesicles or punched out lesions typical of a herpes infection.

Emollients are crucial to moisturize the skin and prevent it drying out and cracking. What preparations might be helpful to Mohammed and how much should you give?

Ointments are better absorbed than creams and good for dry scaly eczema. A soothing emollient is a 50/50 mixture of soft paraffin and oily cream. Much more expensive and not currently on prescription are the oatmeal-based creams (such as Aveeno). It is important that Mrs Begum does not use soap on Mohammed's skin as the detergent may cause irritation and drying. You could prescribe a different bath oil and suggest she uses the aqueous cream instead of soap to cleanse the skin gently and then applies the soft paraffin and oily cream afterwards.

Mrs Begum asks you if Mohammed might have a food allergy that is causing the eczema and wonders if she should be taking him off dairy products.

Only about 10% of children are thought to be sensitive to foods that make their eczema worse, but as Mrs Begum has raised the issue of diet and you have noticed that Mohammed is quite overweight, you should find out what she is giving him to eat and drink.

Mrs Begum tells you that he is still taking a bottle and has four or five 8-oz bottles of milk a day, plus she likes to 'treat' him with sweets and a fizzy drink when the other children come in from school. He eats some fruit and meat and rice.

What daily intake of milk is recommended for toddlers?

By the age of 2 years a child does not need more than half a pint (10 fl oz) of cow's milk a day so Mohammed is having much more than he needs. This may partly account for his increased weight. Some fizzy drinks contain tartrazine (a food colouring) which may make eczema worse in some children. Sweets are likely to lead to tooth decay as well as causing weight gain.

You suggest gently to Mrs Begum that it would be much better for Mohammed's health to reduce his milk intake and increase the amount of fruit and vegetables in his diet. You ask her to bring Mohammed to the baby clinic for weighing and to see the health visitor for further dietary advice.

You are going to give Mohammed some oral antibiotics but is it worth also using topical steroid and/or antibiotic creams?

When the skin is acutely inflamed and infected, a short course of a combined steroid and antibiotic cream such as Fucibet or Fucidin H may be appropriate if the skin is not broken. In Mohammed's case, you may want to give Mrs Begum a small amount of hydrocortisone 1% ointment to use once a day on any very inflamed patches of skin, as well as the oral antibiotics and emollients.

It is always advisable to use the least potent steroid that will control the eczema and advise the parent to apply it for up to a week. Very potent steroids should not be used for children with atopic eczema in primary care (Table 6).

What are you going to say to Mrs Begum and what practical tips can you give her?

• Reassure her that you can help Mohammed with his eczema
• Her role is crucial in keeping his skin moisturized (at least four times a day)
• He should not have too much bedding at night
• Cotton clothing is preferable to synthetic materials (which tend to be hotter)
• She should cut his nails short so he cannot scratch so easily

It is also important that he takes the full 2-week course of antibiotic medicine. You explain to Mrs Begum that eczema is a condition that comes and goes with intermittent flare-ups. She should make sure she always has sufficient supplies of creams and ointments to treat Mohammed when his skin deteriorates. She will need approximately 250 g/week of emollients. The National

Table 6 Topical steroids.

Very potent	Clobetasol propionate 0.05% (Dermovate)
Potent	Mometasone furoate 0.1% (Elocon) Fluticasone proprionate 0.05% (Cutivate)
Moderately potent	Clobetasol butyrate 0.05% (Eumovate)
Mild	Hydrocortisone 1% & 0.5%

Eczema Society produces excellent fact sheets for patients and carers on management of eczema so you may want to give Mrs Begum their address and contact details (National Eczema Society, Hill House, Highgate Hill, London N19 5NA. Tel: 020 7281 3553. Helpline: 0870 241 3604. www.eczema.org).

You give Mrs Begum the prescription for flucloxacillin 125 mg q.i.d. for 2 weeks, a 500-g tub of 50/50 soft paraffin and oily cream and ask her to make another appointment to see you in a few days. She says she will bring Mohammed to the next baby clinic for weighing.

What follow-up is appropriate?

You should offer to see Mohammed in 5–7 days to make sure he is improving. At this next appointment, you should talk to Mrs Begum about the use of mild topical steroids for treating flare-ups of the eczema. You should also contact the health visitor to ask her to see Mohammed regularly for weighing and dietary advice.

Referral to secondary care should be considered if Mohammed still has obvious infected eczema when you next see him despite the treatment you have prescribed.

What other treatments have you heard about that are very effective for bad childhood eczema?

You may have heard of 'wet wraps'. This is a technique that can be taught to parents, usually by a nurse in the dermatology clinic or a practice nurse who has experience of treating childhood eczema. Tubular cotton bandages and vests are used to cover the skin after moisturization and steroid creams have been applied. The first layer of bandages are soaked in water and squeezed dry before being rolled on to moisturized skin so they remain slightly moist. A second layer of dry bandages are then applied to keep the others in place. The bandages help to soothe the hot dry skin and prevent the child scratching and are usually used only at night.

Topical tacrolimus and pimecrolimus are relatively new topical treatments which are used for moderate to severe eczema in adults and children aged 2 years and older which has not been controlled by topical steroids. It is recommended that treatment with these should be initiated only by physicians and GPs with a special interest and experience in dermatology.

PART 2: CASES

CASE REVIEW

Mohammed's case presents a common scenario of a miserable feverish child and an anxious exhausted parent. It is important that Mrs Begum understands that atopic eczema is a common relapsing condition and cannot be cured. However, she can do a great deal to keep the problem under control by using moisturizers regularly (3–4 times a day) and topical steroids for short periods for any flare-ups of the condition. It is also essential that she recognizes when to seek medical help if Mohammed's eczema becomes crusty or weepy, so any skin infection can be treated promptly. The support of the health visitor should be enlisted in reinforcing the message about moisturization and in giving advice about Mohammed's diet and weight. Simple recommendations about clothing, avoidance of irritants such as biological washing powders and soap and making sure Mohammed does not get too hot can also be mentioned.

Atopic eczema is very common and affects 15–20% of schoolchildren and 2–10% of adults in the UK (Patient Information Leaflet – Eczema atopic. Prodigy website www.cks.library.nhs.uk/eczema_atopic/patient_information). It usually manifests itself before the age of 1

year. The aetiology is not fully understood but is probably related to a mixture of genetic and environmental factors. It is associated with other atopic conditions such as asthma and hayfever and there is a family history in 67% of cases. It often improves by puberty.

The red rash is caused by intracellular oedema and white cell infiltrates in the dermis and high serum levels of immunoglobulin E (IgE) have been noted in 80% of people with atopic eczema. Irritants such as detergents, soaps and some chemicals can trigger eczema and extremes of temperature and humidity may also have a role.

According to NICE guidelines (2004), emollients are the first line treatment for atopic eczema and help retain the skin's barrier function and prevent painful cracking. Topical steroids should be used when the eczema is inflamed for short periods of time and in the lowest strength appropriate for the severity of the disease, to minimize the side effects such as skin thinning.

There is some controversy in the literature about the avoidance of allergens. A systematic review by Hoare *et al.* (2000) of atopic eczema stated that there was no randomized controlled trial evidence to show the clinical benefit of

Continued

avoiding enzyme washing powders, wearing cotton clothing as opposed to soft-weave synthetics and applying twice-daily as opposed to once-daily topical corticosteroids, topical antibiotic/steroid combinations versus topical steroids alone or antiseptic bath additives. However, there is plenty of anecdotal evidence to suggest that some children are either sensitive to detergents, or their eczema is irritated by exposure to these. Cotton clothing is cooler than synthetic fabrics and less likely to adhere to the skin.

Mohammed is an overweight child which will exacerbate his eczema. His father, Mr Khan (who appears elsewhere in this book) also has health problems partly related to his weight. It is a challenge but extremely worthwhile to try and encourage Mrs Begum to improve Mohammed's diet and reduce his calorie intake, both to improve his skin and to try and prevent long-term health risks such as diabetes.

KEY POINTS

- Moisturization is the key to controlling the scratch–itch cycle. Parents need instruction about frequency and amounts to apply
- Topical steroids should be used for flare-ups of the eczema in the least potent preparation that will control the problem. Once daily applications are usually sufficient
- Bacterial infections commonly cause exacerbations (usually caused by *Staphylococcus aureus*) and are evident by crusting and exudation and should be treated promptly with a 2-week course of systemic antibiotics
- Simple measures such as wearing cotton clothing, cutting the nails and wearing mittens at night can help prevent scratching
- Food allergies are an uncommon cause of eczema. If sensitivity to certain foods seems likely, referral to a dietitian might be appropriate
- Referral to a paediatric dermatologist may be necessary if the eczema is severe and resistant to treatment

References

British National Formulary. (2007) British Medical Association and the Royal Pharmaceutical Association of Great Britain, London.

Hoare, C., Li Wan Po, A. & Williams, H. (2000) Systematic review of treatments for atopic eczema. *Health Technology Assessment* **4**, 1–191. http://www.ncchta.org/exec-summ/summ437.htm Accessed on 21 July 2007.

National Institute for Health and Clinical Excellence (NICE). (2004) *Atopic dermatitis (eczema) – topical steroids.* Technology Appraisal Guidance No. 81. http://www.guidance.nice.org.uk/TA81/guidance/pdf/English/download.dspx Accessed on 21 July 2007.

Patient Information Leaflet, Eczema atopic. http://www.cks.library.nhs.uk/eczema_atopic/patient_information Accessed on 28 November 2007.

Primary Care Dermatology Society. http://www.pcds.org.uk/Information%20Resource/Guide_manatopic.asp Accessed on 22 July 2007.

Prodigy guidance. *Atopic eczema.* http://www.cks.library.nhs.uk/eczema_atopic/in_depth Accessed on 21 July 2007.

A 17-year-old man with rash and fever

You are the duty doctor on call for a busy practice. One of your duties is to triage telephone calls. You are called by Pip who is concerned about her 17-year-old boyfriend, Pete. He is in bed with what they thought was flu as it is 'going round at the moment' but she is now worried as he is rapidly getting worse. He is unable to get out of bed, as he is so weak, with aching joints and dizziness. She also says that he is 'burning up' and on stripping him off to cool him down she has noticed that he has developed a red rash.

You do not know either Pip or Pete but they are both patients on your list.

What is the diagnosis that needs to be ruled out?

In all presentations to general practice you should try and rule out the most serious conditions first, in this case meningococcal septicaemia.

What type of rash would increase your suspicion of meningococcal septicaemia and how should it be assessed?

A non-blanching rash, assessed by the glass test. This involves pressing a glass firmly against the rash to see if it fades under pressure.

Pip says that her mum told her how to do the test and she has done it already. She was reassured by the fact that the rash faded under pressure.

Is she right to be reassured?

It should be remembered that up to 11% of children with a petechial rash will have meningococcal disease but up to 30% of children with meningococcal disease will present with a non-specific maculopapular rash (Plate 4, facing p. 56). Differentiating between a maculopapular viral rash and maculopapular meningococcal rash is impossible (Hart & Thomson 2006).

What are your management options?

You need to triage the call and decide whether to:
- Call for an ambulance
- Visit Pete at home immediately
- Visit after morning surgery
- Ask them to come in to see you

From the information that you have, you cannot rule out meningococcal septicaemia and so you decide to visit immediately as you need to quickly determine the diagnosis and arrange management accordingly.

Meningococcal septicaemia can be fatal and every minute delay in treatment is crucial (Hahne *et al.* 2006). Before you go you need to make sure that you have benzylpenicillin as this is the correct initial 'blind therapy' if meningococcal disease is suspected. It comes in a powder and so you will also need water for reconstitution in your medical bag.

What are the symptoms and signs that you should look for that would indicate meningitis or meningococcal septicaemia?

See Box 25 and Box 26.

When you arrive you confirm that Pete has been unwell for less than 24 h. On examination he is fully conscious, flushed, has a temperature of 39.2°, pulse rate 106 beats/min, BP 102/65 mmHg. He has a headache and is not photophobic but is a little phonophobic. He has a maculopapular rash but has three non-blanching spots on his chest. There is no neck stiffness.

What is the most important thing to do next?

You should arrange for urgent hospital admission as Pete's history and the examination findings confirm your suspicions of meningococcal infection.

Box 25 Meningitis symptoms

Department of Health (2006).

In babies

- A high pitched moaning cry
- Irritable when picked up
- A bulging fontanelle
- Drowsy and less responsive
- Floppy and restless or stiff with jerky movements
- Refusing feeds
- Vomiting
- Skin that is pale, blotchy, or turning blue
- Fever

In older children

- A stiff neck
- A very bad headache
- Dislike of bright lights
- Vomiting
- Fever
- Drowsy or confused
- Rash

Box 26 Septicaemia symptoms

Department of Health (2006).

In babies

- Rapid or unusual pattern of breathing
- Skin that is pale, blotchy or turning blue
- Fever with cold hands and feet
- Shivering
- Vomiting or refusal to feed
- Red or purple spots that do not fade under pressure
- Pain/irritability from muscle pain or severe limb/joint pain
- Floppiness
- Severe sleepiness

In older children

- Sleepiness or confusion
- Severe pain and aches in joint and limbs
- Very cold hands and feet
- Shivering
- Rapid breathing
- Red or purple spots that do not fade under pressure
- Vomiting
- Fever
- Diarrhoea and stomach cramps

Should you give any treatment before he is admitted?

The evidence for pre-admission antibiotics being beneficial is still under debate (Hahne *et al.* 2006; Keeley 2006) but the Department of Health advice for a non-blanching rash with some of the symptoms listed above is that it is indicative of meningococcal septicaemia and therefore antibiotics should be given immediately and rapid hospital admission arranged (Box 27; Department of Health 2006; HPA Meningococcus Forum 2006).

Box 27 Blind therapy for meningococcal septicaemia

BNF (2006).

- Benzylpenicillin should be given by intravenous or intramuscular injection at the dose of 1.2 g
- You should check for any allergies prior to administering any medication
- Cefotaxime if the patient is penicillin allergic

If your index of suspicion of meningococcal disease is very low, rapid admission for assessment and treatment without pre-hospital parenteral antibiotics may be more appropriate as antibacterial culture is more likely to be successful if antibiotics have not been given (Moller & Skinhoj 2000).

When you ask if he has any allergies Pete says that he is allergic to penicillin.

Is this sufficient evidence to prevent you giving the benzylpenicillin?

No. You need to ask him some more questions as many people incorrectly think that they have an allergy when they do not. This is because many members of the general public are unable to distinguish between symptoms that are caused by side-effects of a medication versus those caused by an allergic reaction.

He says that a course of penicillin given to him for a sore throat as a child gave him diarrhoea and on further questioning he had no symptoms to indicate an allergic reaction. You therefore decide to give the dose of benzylpenicillin and arrange for an ambulance to admit Pete to hospital urgently.

The diagnosis of meningococcal septicaemia is confirmed. He is treated with a course of intravenous benzylpenicillin and is discharged home a couple of weeks later without any complications.

A few days later you get a call from a friend who sits next to Pete at college. He is worried as he has heard that Pete has been admitted to hospital and has been told that he needs antibiotics.

How should you respond?

Although the communicable diseases control team will deal with prophylaxis of patient contacts you still have a duty to answer concerns of the friends and family about their exposure to the index case.

Who should receive prophylaxis?

See Box 28.

Box 28 Chemoprophylaxis

- Should be given to the following two groups:
  - prolonged close contact during the 7 days prior to the onset of the illness
  - transient contact but been exposed to large particle droplets/secretions from the respiratory tract of the index case around the time of admission to hospital
- Should be given as soon as possible, preferably within 24 h (HPA Meningococcus Forum 2006)
- The antibiotics used are rifampicin or ciprofloxacin (*BNF* 2006).

You confirm with the friend that they do not belong to either of the two categories and so do not need prophylaxis.

How do you reassure him?

You reassure him that most cases of the disease are isolated cases. Also you say that transient contact with a case is unlikely to be a risk factor to developing the disease and the risk even to members of the same household is small. It is also now a considerable time since Pete became unwell and the incubation period is usually 3–5 days.

Is this where your duty ends?

You also have an ongoing duty to ensure that your population base receives the current recommended vaccination programme, which includes meningococcal C vaccination (Box 29). Full details of the routine immunization programme can be found in the Appendix.

All cases of suspected meningococcal infection should be reported to the communicable diseases control team without waiting for a definitive diagnosis (HPA Meningococcus Forum 2006). The list of other notifiable dis-

---

Box 29 Meningococcal C vaccination

- All children starting their immunization programme receive meningitis C immunization at 3, 4 and 12 months old
- Children too old to receive the primary vaccination programme are given a catch-up programme

---

eases, under the Public Health Regulations 1988, includes food poisoning, measles and tuberculosis. This list can be found on the Health Protection Agency website (www.hpa.org).

CASE REVIEW

This case highlights the importance of having an appropriate triage system in place. Telephone consultations are useful but are not a substitute for a home visit, particularly in an emergency situation. Even if an ambulance is going to be called it is important to attend so that you can fully assess the patient as this will enable you to give a clear referral to the hospital, to administer immediately necessary treatment and to offer support to the patient and family.

GPs are fearful of meningococcal disease. Research states that it is difficult to reach a diagnosis and that half of children with meningococcal disease are sent home at the first primary care consultation (Brennan *et al.* 2003; Harnden 2007). The diagnostic difficulties outlined by Harnden include the fact the serious bacterial infection is rare, that early symptoms can mimic common and self-limiting viral infections, measurement of vital signs can be difficult in children and to help overcome these difficulties we should be prepared to offer a full clinical assessment by an experienced clinician to all feverish children. You therefore need to be clear of the symptoms and signs to look out for.

Neisseria meningitidis is a normal inhabitant of the nasopharynx and is spread by droplet secretion (Cartwright 1995). Most individuals who carry the bacteria do not progress to invasive disease and most cases involve the B or C serotypes. Invasive disease presents as septicaemia, meningitis, or both (HPA Meningococcus Forum 2006).

Continued

PART 2: CASES

An immunization programme for meningitis C was brought in to help combat the rising number of cases in the UK, 40% of which are caused by meningitis C. It should be noted that the rest are caused by meningitis B for which there is still no vaccine. The number of laboratory confirmed cases of meningitis C has dropped 90% since the introduction of the vaccine and only accounts for 10% of the cases of meningococcal disease (Department of Health 2006).

KEY POINTS

- *N. meningitidis* is a normal inhabitant of the nasopharynx
- Invasive disease presents as meningitis, septicaemia, or both
- Meningococcal septicaemia does not necessarily present with a petechial rash
- Initial blind therapy is benzylpenicillin or cefotaxime if penicillin allergic
- There is a UK vaccination programme for meningitis C
- Meningococcal septicaemia is a notifiable disease
- Prophylactic antibiotics should be given to the following two groups:
  - prolonged close contact during the 7 days prior to the onset of the illness
  - those who have had transient contact but been exposed to large particle droplets/secretions from the respiratory tract of the index case around the time of admission to hospital

References

Brennan, C.A., Somerset, M., Granier, S.K., Fahey T.P. & Heyderman R.S. (2003) Management of diagnostic uncertainty in children with possible meningitis: a qualitative study. *British Journal of General Practice* **53**, 626–631.

British National Formulary, 52nd edn. (2006) Royal Pharmaceutical Society of Great Britain. RPS Publishing and BMJ Publishing Group, London.

Cartwright, K.A.V. (1995) *Meningococcal Disease.* John Wiley and Sons, Chichester.

Department of Health, Chief Medical Officer. (2006) *Preventing meningitis.* http://www.doh.gov.uk/en/Aboutus/MinistersandDepartmentLeaders/ChiefMedicalOfficer/ProgressonPolicy/ProgressBrowsableDocument/DH_4102778 Accessed on 14 February 2007.

Hahne, S.J.M., Charlett, A., Purcell, B., *et al.* (2006) Effectiveness of antibiotics given before admission in reducing mortality from meningococcal disease: systematic review. *BMJ* **332**, 1299–1303.

Harnden, A. (2007) Recognising serious illness in feverish young children in primary care. *BMJ* **335**, 409–410.

Hart, C.A. & Thomson, A.P.J. (2006) Meningococcal disease and its management in children. *BMJ* **333**, 685–90.

Health Protection Agency (HPA) Meningococcus Forum. (2006) *Guidance for public health management of meningococcal disease in the UK.* http://hpa.org.uk/infections/topics_az/meningococcalguidelines.pdf Accessed on 14 February 2007.

Keeley, D. (2006) Parenteral penicillin before admission to hospital for meningitis. *BMJ* **332**, 1283–1284.

Moller, K. & Skinhoj, P. (2000) Guidelines for managing acute bacterial meningitis. *BMJ* **320**, 1290.

Newell, S.J. & Darling, J.C. (2008) *Lecture Notes: Paediatrics,* 8th edn. Blackwell Publishing, Oxford.

Case 14   A 46-year-old man with indigestion

Mr Johnson, a 46-year-old scaffolder, comes to the surgery complaining of pain in the upper abdomen after eating, intermittent heartburn, bloating and excessive wind. This has been going on for about 2 months and is getting worse. Mr Johnson's records show he attends the surgery rarely and you have not seen him before.

What immediate diagnoses spring to mind?

• Non-ulcer functional dyspepsia or gastritis (many different causes including alcohol, *Helicobacter pylori* infection and non-steroidal anti-inflammatory drugs [NSAIDs])
• Peptic ulcer (could be idiopathic or caused by NSAIDs or *H. pylori* infection)
• Gastro-oesophageal reflux disease (GORD)
• Upper gastrointestinal cancer

What specific questions do you need to ask to find out more about his symptoms?

• Are there any foods that make the problem worse?
• Any difficulty swallowing?
• Has he had any vomiting?
• Has he lost any weight?
• Any change in his appetite?
• Has he passed any black motions?
• Does he wake at night with the pain?

Mr Johnson tells you that he has not noticed that any particular foods make the problem worse. Swallowing is fine and he has not vomited but has felt nauseated sometimes and this is happening more frequently recently. His appetite is unchanged and he does not think he has lost weight. His motions are normal. He has woken up a few times at night with pain and usually gets up for a drink of milk.

What other lifestyle questions are important?

• Does he smoke or drink alcohol?
• Is he on any regular medications or over-the-counter remedies?

• Has he tried any treatments himself?
• What does he think might be the problem?

He is a non-smoker but drinks 2–3 pints of beer at night, more at weekends and occasionally a whisky. He takes ibuprofen 400 mg t.i.d. for a chronic back problem and co-codamol intermittently. He has tried some Rennies (antacid containing calcium carbonate, magnesium carbonate and sodium alginate), which helped a bit. He is not sure what the problem might be but wondered if he was developing an ulcer.

Any other relevant information?

• Family history of peptic ulcer
• Family history of upper gastrointestinal cancer
• Past history of Barrett's oesophagus or pernicious anaemia
• General past medical history

Mr Johnson had a back injury 10 years ago after falling off scaffolding. He has chronic low back pain for which he has been prescribed various analgesics over the years, but finds ibuprofen is the most useful. He has been taking this with occasional co-codamol for the last 4 years. He has no history of previous problems with indigestion.

There is no family history of either cancer or peptic ulcer.

When you come to examine Mr Johnson, apart from being slightly overweight with a body mass index (BMI) of 27, and slight tenderness in the upper epigastrium, physical examination is normal.

Looking back at your original list of differential diagnoses, what seems the most likely choices and why?

• *Non-ulcer functional dyspepsia or gastritis:* quite likely as he is drinking more than the recommended amount of alcohol and taking NSAIDs, both of which are irritant to the gastric mucosa
• *Peptic ulcer:* also likely as he has pain at night and has been taking NSAIDs for several years, but there is no family history or previous problems

• *GORD:* possible, but no history of acid taste in mouth, substernal pain or symptoms worsening on lying flat

• *Upper gastrointestinal cancer:* not sounding very likely as he has no 'alarm symptoms' or Red flags

---

!RED FLAG

Patients with dyspepsia with any of the following should be referred urgently for endoscopy:

• Progressive dysphagia
• Unintentional weight loss
• Iron deficiency anaemia
• Persistent vomiting
• Epigastric mass
• Gastrointestinal bleed (ask about vomiting up blood or passing black tarry stools – melaena)

NICE guidelines also recommend that patients aged 55 years and over should be referred urgently for endoscopy if dyspepsia symptoms are:

• Recent in onset rather than recurrent
• Unexplained
• Persistent for more than 4–6 weeks

What do you do next?

You decide to arrange a blood test to exclude anaemia (and possibly liver function tests and a gamma glutamyl transferase [GGT] test because you are worried that his alcohol intake may be much higher than he is admitting – most people tend to underestimate).

You advise him to stop taking the ibuprofen and any other NSAIDs including aspirin (paracetamol is a good alternative). You also mention that he should reduce his alcohol intake to no more than 21 units/week (1.5 pints/day beer) and avoid spirits and caffeine. Fatty and very spicy foods can make indigestion worse so grill rather than fry and eat lean meat, fresh vegetables and avoid hot curries.

Mr Johnson is willing to stop taking the ibuprofen if you give him co-codamol instead, but is less keen to reduce his alcohol intake or change his diet. He goes to see the practice nurse for the blood tests.

What other strategies might be helpful?

Find out who does the shopping and cooking in the household and offer to see them with Mr J. to discuss dietary changes.

Enlist the support of an interested practice nurse and/or community dietitian.

Does he need an endoscopy or a test for *H. pylori*?

If his blood tests are normal and there are no Red flag symptoms or signs, NICE guidelines state that: 'Routine endoscopic investigation of patients of any age, presenting with dyspepsia and without alarm signs, is not necessary.'

The guidelines also say that there is insufficient evidence to conclude whether it is better to treat simple dyspepsia without investigating further at this stage or whether to test for *H. pylori* and treat if positive.

Mr Johnson is not keen to have many tests and investigations and prefers to try some treatment first.

What treatment would be suitable and how long should it be given for?

Antacids such as Gaviscon liquid 5–10 mL as required or 1–2 tablets chewed after meals (Gaviscon contains sodium alginate, sodium bicarbonate and calcium carbonate)

As Mr Johnson's symptoms are deteriorating and gastritis or an ulcer seems possible, it would be wise to also give:

• A proton pump inhibitor (PPI) such as omeprazole 20 mg or lansoprazole 30 mg o.d. for 4–8 weeks; or

• An H_2-histamine receptor antagonist (H_2RA) such as cimetidine 400 mg b.i.d. for 4 weeks

PPIs are more effective than H_2RAs at reducing dyspeptic symptoms in trials of patients with uninvestigated dyspepsia.

What do you say to Mr Johnson about the treatment and follow-up?

You reassure him that even if he does have an ulcer, tablets can be used to heal this up and that he is likely to get better if he follows your lifestyle advice and takes the prescribed medication for a minimum of 4 weeks. His indigestion may be caused by irritation of the stomach lining, made worse by alcohol and tablets such as ibuprofen. You want to see him again in 3–4 weeks after giving him a prescription for an antacid, a PPI and co-codamol for his back pain. If he is no better at that stage, you might need to arrange some other investigations.

Follow-up

Mr Johnson's blood tests are normal apart from a slightly raised GGT of 73 IU/L (normal 0–51 IU/L) which is probably brought about by his alcohol consumption.

Four weeks later Mr Johnson reappears and unfortunately he is still symptomatic. He says he has cut the drinking down 'a bit', stopped the ibuprofen and is taking the Gaviscon and PPI, but he still has problems with bloating and pain in the upper abdomen after eating. He is also constipated with the co-codamol you gave him and finds it less effective for his back problem than the ibuprofen.

What do you do next?

Codeine-based analgesics often cause constipation. You could prescribe a laxative such as lactulose and advise him to increase the fibre in his diet. Although there are combined preparations of NSAIDs with a synthetic prostaglandin analogue with antisecretory and protective properties (e.g. Arthrotec = diclofenac plus misoprostol), it would not be advisable to prescribe this because he is still symptomatic.

You decide that you need to rule out *H. pylori* infection, which could also be contributing to his symptoms.

How do you arrange this and what do you tell Mr Johnson?

Helicobacter pylori can be initially detected using a carbon-13 urea breath test, a stool antigen test or a blood test. Which you choose will depend on local availability and preferences.

A 2-week washout period following PPI use is necessary before testing for *H. pylori* with a breath test or a stool antigen test.

In your practice, breath tests are commonly used but it can take several weeks to arrange one. You tell Mr Johnson that you will organize this and when he receives the appointment, he needs to stop taking his PPI 2 weeks before the test.

Doctors are sometimes guilty of not explaining to patients what a test actually entails, whether it is uncomfortable and how long it takes. You should tell Mr Johnson about the breath test (Box 30).

When should you see Mr Johnson again after the breath test?

It may take at least a week for the breath test result to be sent to you so you ask Mr Johnson to make another appointment 7–10 days after he has had the test so that you can give him the result and prescribe treatment if necessary. He can restart the PPI after the breath test while he is waiting to see you again.

> **Box 30 Breath test for *Helicobacter pylori***
>
> *Helicobacter pylori* is a bacteria that is found commonly in the stomach and can cause ulceration and symptoms of indigestion. It can be eradicated by taking tablets. A simple way to detect the presence of the bacteria is a 'breath test' in which a sample of your breath is taken by asking you to blow into a balloon or blow bubbles into a bottle of liquid. You will then be given a capsule or some water to swallow that contains urea tagged with a special type of carbon. This is not harmful but may taste nasty.
>
> Samples of your breath will then be collected periodically after swallowing the urea. The breath sample will be tested to determine whether it contains the tagged carbon (resulting from the breakdown of the urea). If it does, the test is positive and you do have *H. pylori* in the stomach.
>
> The urea breath test usually takes about 1.5 h.

Six weeks later Mr Johnson's breath test comes back as positive for *H. pylori*. What treatment are you going to prescribe?

Helicobacter pylori eradication requires a combination of two antibiotics and PPIs. There are various therapy regimens lasting 7–14 days which are listed in the *British National Formulary* (*BNF*) including:

Regimen 1
- Clarithromycin 500 mg b.i.d.
- Amoxicillin 1 g b.i.d.
- Omeprazole 20 mg b.i.d.

or

Regimen 2
- Metronidazole 400 mg b.i.d.
- Clarithromycin 500 mg b.i.d.
- Omeprazole 20 mg b.i.d.

You check with Mr Johnson to make sure he is not allergic to any medications before prescribing him the first regimen.

It can be very difficult to take so many medications every day (6 or more tablets twice a day) so you need to encourage Mr Johnson to try and complete the course. You warn him that the antibiotics can cause diarrhoea and nausea, but this might help his constipation temporarily.

Outcome. Two weeks later Mr Johnson comes back to see you and this time his indigestion is much better. He asks if he has to continue taking tablets.

You could try stopping the PPI and just continuing with the antacid as and when he needs it. However, in some patients, when they stop the PPI they become symptomatic again so they tend to go on a long-term maintenance dose (the lowest possible, e.g. omeprazole 10 mg/day or lansoprazole 15 mg/day). Mr Johnson is keen to come off regular medication so you agree to prescribe him just an antacid at the moment but ask him to come back to see you if his symptoms return. You also advise him again about limiting his alcohol intake as this is likely to exacerbate his indigestion and damage his liver.

CASE REVIEW

Indigestion or dyspepsia is a common presentation in general practice (3–4% of consultations) and it is not appropriate to investigate or treat all cases. As in Mr Johnson's case, it is important to take a good history, identify any factors that may be contributing to the problem such as alcohol and medications (self-care or prescribed) and give advice about modifying any factors that may be exacerbating the problem. Most cases of dyspepsia are not caused by cancer, but any of the Red flag symptoms mentioned, particularly in those over 55 years, should lead to immediate investigation and prompt referral.

Mr Johnson had been taking ibuprofen for many years for a back problem. Other analgesics besides NSAIDs should be offered if it is thought they are causing the indigestion. An alert should be added to his notes that he should not be prescribed NSAIDs in the future.

It is over 20 years since the association of *H. pylori* with peptic ulceration was first recognized. *H. pylori* is associated with >90% of duodenal ulcers and >80% of gastric ulcers and may have a role in the development of gastric cancer, although a causal relationship has not been proven. Testing for the bacterium and treating it with 'triple therapy' need careful explanation to the patient in order for them to understand and comply with any procedures such as breath testing and concord with the large quantity of tablets they will have to take if the test is positive.

According to the *BNF*, NSAID use and *H. pylori* infection are independent risk factors for gastrointestinal bleeding and ulceration and it is not entirely clear in Mr Johnson's case whether both contributed to his symptoms or just one of them.

KEY POINTS

Indigestion or dyspepsia is common. In the UK this is caused by (NPC 2006):
- Non-ulcer or functional dyspepsia (40%)
- Peptic ulcer disease (13%)
- Gastro-oesophageal reflux disease (40%)
- Upper gastrointestinal cancers (<2%) – less than 1 in 1 million under-55-year-olds with dyspepsia have cancer
- Endoscopic biopsy, breath tests and serology all have sensitivities and specificities >90%
- Serology remains positive for up to 9 months after eradication
- Breath tests become negative with *H. pylori* eradication and are therefore used to confirm eradication if appropriate

Finally, if Mr Johnson's symptoms recurred or continued despite treatment, referral for a gastroenterological opinion would be appropriate and he should have an endoscopy.

References

British National Formulary. (March, 2006) British Medical Association and Royal Pharmaceutical Society of Great Britain BMJ Publishing Group Ltd London.

National Institute for Health and Clinical Excellence (NICE). (2004) *Dyspepsia: management of dyspepsia in adults in primary care.* Clinical guideline No. 17. http://www.nice.org.uk Accessed on 23 February 2008.

The National Prescribing Centre. (2006) *The initial management of dyspepsia in primary care.* MeReC Briefing Issue No. 32. www.npc.co.uk/MeReC_briefings/2006/dyspepsia_briefings_no_32.pdf Accessed on 23 February 2008.

An 8-year-old child with abdominal pain

Gillian, aged 8 years, attends the surgery with her father. She refused to go to school for several days during the last term, complaining of several ailments but usually of 'tummy pain'.

Her mother and father had initially thought that this was just an attempt by her to get out of school, particularly as she had only complained during the week and not at weekends. On each of these occasions the symptoms resolved without any treatment.

During the last few days they have been more concerned. She has been complaining of tummy pain again but she has also been off her food and generally 'off colour'.

What are the diagnoses that you need to consider?
- Urinary tract infection
- School refusal
- Recurrent abdominal pain – cause unknown (used to be called periodic syndrome)
- Sexual abuse

What further questions would you like to ask Gillian and her father
Remember that she is old enough to answer some questions herself.
- What has the tummy pain been like?
- Has she had problems like this prior to the last few weeks?
- Has she had any problems with diarrhoea or constipation?
- Has she had any burning when she urinates, been needing to go more often or had any accidents if she has not made it to the toilet?
- How is Gillian getting on at school? Is she missing her friends in the time that she has had off?

Gillian says that her tummy has been aching and that nothing makes it better. She has not had any diarrhoea or

constipation. She has been weeing more often during the last couple of days and her father says that it 'smells strong'. She has had urinary urgency and this caused her to wet her pants on one occasion as she could not get to the bathroom quickly enough. She was very upset about this.

Gillian is getting on fine at school but has been missing her friend Fiona since she has been off.

What is the most likely diagnosis?
Urinary tract infection but you need some more information to confirm the diagnosis.

What are the symptoms of urinary tract infection?
See Box 31.

Box 31 UTI symptoms can be unclear they can include

Prodigy (2005), NICE (2007).
- Pyrexia of unknown origin
- Feeding disorders
- Slow weight gain
- Vomiting
- Diarrhoea
- Sepsis
- General malaise/lethargy
- Prolonged jaundice in the neonate
- Abdominal pain
- Haematuria
- Offensive urine
- Changes to continence

How could you obtain more information to help you to make a diagnosis?
By carrying out an examination:
- General appearance – including pulse and temperature
- Abdominal palpation

PART 2: CASES

- External genitalia examination
- Urinalysis

How can you put her at her ease during examination?

Talk to her. Say that her Daddy can remain with her at all times. Explain that you will have to press on her tummy but that she can tell you to stop at any time if it hurts.

On examination, Gillian looks well, is apyrexial and has no abnormal findings on abdominal or external genitalia examination.

How should you explain how to obtain a urine sample?

Children as old as Gillian can provide a mid-stream urine (MSU) sample. You advise her to urinate a little over the toilet and after the first bit try to catch the middle bit of urine in a container that has been sterilized with boiling water. This should then been transferred into a sample bottle that you will give to them. Advise the parents to refrigerate the specimen unless they are bringing it immediately to the surgery.

In infants, try to get a clean catch specimen (a good tip for this is to try to obtain it in the bath as infants often urinate there). Using a potty to obtain a sample will increase the risk of contamination.

Which are the most important indicators of infection on urine dipstick?

See Box 32.

> **Box 32 Interpreting urinalysis for urinary tract infection**
>
> Huicho *et al.* (2002); Giddens and Robinson (1998); Gorelick and Shaw (1999).
> - Positive leucocytes and positive nitrites has a positive predicted value for UTI of 95%
> - Negative leucocytes and negative nitrites has a negative predictive value of 95%
> - Nitrites can be negative even with a UTI due to short contact time of urine with bacteria due to urinary frequency
> - Care must be taken as false positives may lead to unnecessary investigations and treatment but false negatives risk renal damage

---

- Leucocytes
- Nitrites

She is able to provide a sample immediately and dipstick analysis is positive for leucocytes and nitrites.

Should you send the urine sample to the laboratory?

This is definitely required in children with an upper urinary tract infection at risk of serious illness, or if they are under 3 years old (NICE 2007).

Should you start antibiotics immediately?

It should be remembered that prompt diagnosis, treatment and investigation are essential to prevent scarring (Gorelick & Shaw 1999). Even one urinary infection for less than 3 days can produce scarring (Dick & Feldman 1996).

Gillian's symptoms and urine examination are highly suggestive of lower urinary tract infection and so you should start antibiotics in accordance with NICE guidelines (2007).

Which antibiotic should be given and for how long?

Trimethoprim, oral cephalosporin, nitrofurantoin or amoxicillin are the first line antibiotics and these should all be given for 3 days depending on local guidance (NICE 2007).

What are you going to say to Gillian and her father about your findings?

You should say that the symptoms and examination show that Gillian has probably got a water infection and this can be serious in children if it is not treated with antibiotics as it can lead to scarring of the kidneys. You therefore want to start her on an antibiotic.

Gillian's father asks if there could be any side-effects from the antibiotics. You explain that this is unlikely but that some children get some sickness and diarrhoea or itching but all other side-effects are extremely rare. You also explain that the risks of her developing a scar on her kidneys from the infection if you do not treat it is much greater than the risk of side-effects. He asks how she 'caught it'.

PART 2: CASES

How should you respond?

You say that the infection is caused by bacteria getting into the urine and that most are caused by those that live in our own gut. This often happens from the bacteria that lie around the back passage and these can travel up into the bladder.

He asks if this is what caused her to wet herself?

You explain that the inflammation caused by the infection can mean that children may suddenly need to go to the toilet without warning and this can lead to them wetting themselves. You also reassure him that this should settle down once it has been treated.

You start Gillian on a course of trimethoprim (children 1 month–18 years 4 mg/kg twice daily [max 200 mg] [BNF for Children 2006]) and send off the MSU sample for microscopy and culture. You advise that you would like to see them towards the end of the week with a further urine sample to check that the antibiotics have worked.

Gillian and her father do not attend the appointment that you make for them.

Why might they have not returned?

They may simply have forgotten or they may not have understood the importance of follow-up.

What could you do?

- Wait for them to attend
- Contact the family by letter or telephone call

By calling the family you can ask them directly why they did not attend. Remember not to be too judgemental as you do not want to scare them off completely.

When you call the mother says that Gillian has been completely well for a couple of days and finished the course of antibiotics. The family therefore did not want to waste your time further.

What should you say to her?

You should say that you are happy that Gillian is now settled and ask for a further urine specimen.

Outcome. Gillian goes on to have recurrent infections. She is therefore placed on prophylactic antibiotics and investigations are initiated by the paediatricians. No abnormalities are found.

KEY POINTS

- Approximately 11.3% of girls and 3.6% of boys will be referred for urinary tract infection by the age of 16 years
- Symptoms can be non-specific in children and so diagnosis should be made by urinalysis
- Trimethoprim, oral cephalosporin, nitrofurantoin or amoxicillin are the first line antibiotics in this age group
- Investigations should be carried out to check for renal tract abnormalities and renal scarring if they have a higher renal tract infection, are less than 6 months old, do not respond to treatment or have recurrent infection

CASE REVIEW

Boys are more susceptible to urinary tract infection before the age of 3 months, after that the incidence is much higher in girls. Approximately 11.3% of girls and 3.6% of boys will be referred for this by the age of 16 (Coulthard *et al.* 1997).

Patients may not come to follow-up as you request and in this case Gillian's parents simply did not want to waste your time. However, follow-up is important to check that her treatment has worked. Vesico-ureteric reflux is found in 1% of normal infants and can lead to renal scarring if the child develops an infection (Jacobson *et al.* 1999). At worst, some children with renal scarring will go on to develop hypertension or chronic renal failure (Verrier-Jones *et al.* 2001). Recurrent infection can also occur (20% of boys and 30% of girls; Jodal 1987). Imaging regimes are complex and are usually initiated by secondary care.

Antibiotic prophylaxis is indicated in recurrent infections or proven vesico-ureteric reflux. It should be started immediately after the initial course of antibiotics until specialist investigation is complete (Larcombe 1999).

References
British National Formulary for Children. (2006) Royal Pharmaceutical Society of Great Britain. RPS Publishing and BMJ Publishing Group, London.

Coulthard, M.G., Lambert, H.J. & Keir, M.J. (1997) Occurrence of renal scars in children after their first referral for urinary tract infection. *BMJ* **315**, 918–919.

Dick, P.T. & Feldman, W. (1996) Routine diagnostic imaging for childhood urinary tract infections: a systematic overview. *Journal of Paediatrics* **128**, 15–22.

Giddens, J. & Robinson, G. (1998) How accurately do patients collect urine samples from their children? A pilot study in general practice. *British Journal of General Practice* **48**, 987–988.

Gorelick, M.H. & Shaw, K.N. (1999) Screening tests for urinary tract infection in children: a meta-analysis. *Pediatrics* **104**, e54.

Huicho, L., Compos-Sanchez, M. & Alamo, C. (2002) Meta-analysis of urine screening tests for determining risk of urinary tract infection in children: CME review article. *Paediatric Infectious Disease Journal* **21**, 1–11.

Jacobson, S.H., Hansson, S. & Jakobsson, B. (1999) Vesico-ureteric reflux: occurrence and long-term risks. *Acta Paediatrica* **88** (Suppl. 431), 22–30.

Jodal, U. (1987) The natural history of bacteriuria in childhood. *Infectious Disease Clinics of North America* **1**, 713–729.

Larcombe, J. (1999) Urinary tract infection in children. *BMJ* **319**, 1173–1175.

National Collaborating Centre for Womens' and Childrens' Health for National Institute for Health and Clinical Excellence. (2007) *Urinary tract infection in children: diagnosis, treatment and long-term management.* RCOG Press, London.

Prodigy guidance. (2005) *UTI: children, UTI (lower) men, UTI (lower) women.* www.cks.library.nhs.uk/clinical_knowledge/clinical_topics/by_alphabet/u Accessed on 11 April 2007.

Verrier-Jones, K., Hockley, B., Scrivener, R., Pollock, J.I., *et al.* (2001) Diagnosis and management of urinary tract infections in children under 2 years: assessment of practice against published guidelines. http://www.rcpch.ac.uk/Research/clinical-Audit/Urinary-Tract-Infections Accessed on 24 March 2008.

A 26-year-old man with abdominal pain

Simon, a young man aged 26, is the son of Nancy (see Case 32). You have not seen Simon since he was 18, when his parents were divorcing and he was experiencing recurrent headaches.

On reviewing his medical record before calling him in, you see that he was seen in accident and emergency with abdominal pain at the weekend and that he had been told to see his GP as soon as possible. He comes in with a young woman whom he introduces as his fiancée, Tina, and they both tell how he had terrific pains and bloating all over his abdomen associated with belching and wind, and that she had rushed him up to the hospital.

What are your immediate thoughts about the possible diagnosis?

- Irritable bowel syndrome
- Crohn's disease
- Acute gastroenteritis
- Coeliac disease
- Bowel obstruction

What further information would be useful?

- Did he have any vomiting or fever?
- Had he eaten any 'fast food' or takeaways prior to the pain coming on?
- How are his bowels? Any constipation or diarrhoea? When did he last open them?
- How are his general health and appetite. Has there been any weight loss?
- Has he had any blood in the motions? Or mucus?
- Has this occurred before?

Simon tells you he had no vomiting or fever and feels back to normal today. He felt better once he opened his bowels properly. His bowels go through phases of being very erratic – sometimes he does not open them for several days and on other days he has diarrhoea several times before going to

work. He has never had any blood in the stools, but sometimes they are mucusy.

His general health is good and he has not lost any weight. He admitted that recently he has not been eating regularly because he and Tina have been very preoccupied with their wedding plans. He has had several bouts of similar abdominal pains over the last few years and they are very worried that there is something seriously wrong.

The above history points towards the diagnosis of irritable bowel syndrome (Box 33).

Box 33 Typical features of irritable bowel syndrome (IBS)

Recurrent symptoms of the following:
- Abdominal pain
- Distension/bloating
- Flatulence and or wind
- Diarrhoea or constipation, sometimes both
- Absence of rectal bleeding or weight loss

Should you examine Simon?

Yes. Although examining Simon is unlikely to give you any additional information, it is important to do it to reassure him and, almost as importantly, his girlfriend. The history Simon has given makes you decide that a rectal examination is unnecessary.

As expected, everything is normal in the examination apart from overactive bowel sounds. When you give him the good news, he is visibly relieved and says that he honestly thought he had cancer. His grandfather died of cancer of the bowel. You explain that inherited cancer (e.g. familial polyposis coli) of the bowel is very rare and that he can put this out of his mind. Tina asks you how you can be so sure there is nothing seriously wrong without doing any tests?

What do you say and do next?

• Offer to do some routine blood tests (Box 34)
• Explain that there are no specific tests to confirm irritable bowel syndrome and that this is the most likely diagnosis
• Briefly explain what irritable bowel syndrome is
• Explain the reasons for each test. Coeliac disease is underdiagnosed and needs to be excluded

---

Box 34 Routine tests

• Full blood count to exclude anaemia, and macrocytosis which could be caused by malabsorption
• Erythrocyte sedimentation rate (ESR) or C-reactive protein to exclude inflammatory bowel disease
• IgA tissue transglutaminase
• Stool sample for culture and sensitivity to exclude bacterial gastroenteritis
• You could consider measuring B_{12} and folate levels too, as additional ways of excluding malabsorption

---

Your 10 min is nearly up, so you give Simon a prescription for mebeverine. You ask him to keep a record of any foods that seem to upset him, to try to eat at regular times and drink at least 2 L of fluids per day. You arrange to see him in 2 weeks for a review and to discuss the results of blood tests.

Why did you choose mebeverine and what is the rationale of drug treatment for irritable bowel syndrome?

See Box 35.

Box 35 Drug treatment for irritable bowel syndrome

Drug treatment should aim to relieve symptoms:

Antispasmodics	Hyoscine
	Mebeverine
	Peppermint oil capsules
Antidiarrhoeal	Loperamide
Constipation	Ispaghula husk
Herbal treatment, soothes pain of inflamed gut	Slippery elm

Two weeks later Simon returns, this time on his own, to discuss his results which are all in the normal range. Unfortunately, his bowels have not been at all good, with intermittent pain and diarrhoea, despite taking mebeverine three times a day before meals. Tina has also been buying him probiotic drinks from the supermarket but this does not seem to have had any impact so far.

What further help can you offer Simon?

• Give adequate explanation of the condition in language he can understand, and supplement explanation with written information
• Address any further underlying fears about the condition
• Identify any triggers and discuss healthy eating
• Identify psychological factors that might be aggravating his symptoms

You explain how the bowel is a muscular organ which, in some people, is sensitive to different triggers. These can be chemical, from certain foods, or states of mind such as stress and anxiety. When Simon has pain, it is because something is making his intestines go into spasm. After a while they relax again and are back to normal.

You give him an information leaflet about irritable bowel syndrome and suggest that he looks at the website of the IBS network, a national self-help group.

Simon asks whether he should be referred to a specialist 'so he can have a telescope put up his backside'. You advise against this for the time being. You explain again that it is very unlikely indeed that there is anything wrong with his bowels and that a colonoscopy would be an unpleasant and unnecessary way of demonstrating this.

Simon has identified that peppers and sweetcorn seem to go straight through him and that chips and burgers make him very bloated and uncomfortable.

When asked how the wedding arrangements are going, he looks stressed and reveals that his mother has refused to come to the wedding because his father is going to be there. In fact, his mother has disappeared off to some health farm or other in India. Simon does not know that you have been treating his mother for a thyroid condition.

What else can you suggest to improve Simon's quality of life?

• Other antispasmodics – individuals respond differently to different medications
• Loperamide, which he can buy over-the-counter to control diarrhoea

• Discuss the effect of stress and anxiety on the bowel. You hope that this will alleviate the fears he still has of major physical illness
• Discuss relaxation therapies such as yoga
• Ask him if he would be interested in seeing a psychologist

Outcome. You do not see Simon again until 1 year later. He and Tina are married and she is expecting a baby. He is worried about her because she is so tired and nauseated. He has had irritable bowel symptoms intermittently and the diarrhoea in the mornings is particularly bad again. This time he asks to see a specialist, because no medication seems to have helped him, and he wonders if there are any new treatments. You agree to a referral.

What do you write in the referral letter?
• Full history of the condition, and what has been tried already
• Enclose copies of investigation results
• Your assessment of food triggers and psychological factors
• What the patient is hoping for

The visit to the gastroenterology clinic turns out to be very helpful. Colonoscopy was not discussed and instead the consultant prescribed a low dose of amitriptyline for Simon to continue for a year. Luckily, Simon is motivated enough to try this and after a year reports that he thinks he has significantly less diarrhoea and pain.

References
Primary Care Society for Gastroenterology. (2001) *Irritable Bowel Syndrome: Guidelines for General Practice* www.pcsg.org.uk
Prodigy guidance. (2005) *Irritable bowel syndrome* www.cks.library.nhs.uk/irritable_bowel_syndrome/in_depth/background_information.

CASE REVIEW

Simon had typical symptoms of irritable bowel syndrome, triggered by stress and anxiety and some foods. The condition was chronic and fluctuating and he learned to cope with it through explanation and support which enabled him to understand the triggers.

He tried several different drug treatments without much benefit, but was helped by a long course of low-dose amitriptyline.

He is likely to continue to have some problems with irritable bowel syndrome.

KEY POINTS

• There is no specific test for irritable bowel syndrome. Investigation should be kept to a minimum once malabsorption and coeliac disease have been excluded
• There is no need for referral to a specialist initially, unless serious disease is suspected or the patient is over 45 years
• Referral can be helpful for extra reassurance, or if usual therapies do not help
• A patient-centred approach and careful explanation is particularly important because each individual responds differently
• There is no cure, but long-term low dose amitriptyline can 're-educate' the bowel by modifying the brain–bowel interaction in some cases
• The GP must preserve confidentiality when seeing different members of the same family

PART 2: CASES

Case 17   A 78-year-old woman with bruising

The district nurse asks you to do a home visit to see Mrs Gibson, a 78-year-old widow living with her son and daughter-in-law in a nearby council house. She has noticed some bruising on Mrs Gibson's forearms, which she is concerned about. The nurse has been visiting every 2 days to change the dressings on a chronic leg ulcer on Mrs Gibson's left shin. You have never met Mrs Gibson before. According to the nurse, she is a fairly independent elderly woman who can dress and wash herself. She goes out to the corner shops and once a week to the social club, but does not do any cooking or household shopping.

Her other medical problems include high blood pressure and late onset asthma. Her current medications are:

- Bendroflumethiazide 2.5 mg o.d.
- Salmeterol (Serevent) inhaler 2 puffs b.i.d.
- Beclometasone inhaler 100 μg per puff, 2 puffs b.i.d.
- Theophylline M/R (Uniphyllin Continus) 200 mg b.i.d.
- Prednisolone 5 mg/day

Before you go to see Mrs Gibson, what common causes of bruising pass through your mind?

- Thin skin in the elderly
- Falls
- Thrombocytopenia
- Liver disease ± alcohol
- Clotting disorders
- Physical abuse
- Drug-related (e.g. warfarin, aspirin, steroids)

Are there any medications that she is on that might be contributing to the problem?

- *Steroids causing skin thinning:* Mrs Gibson is on a small dose of prednisolone for her asthma
- *Antihypertensive agents:* Mrs Gibson is on bendroflumethiazide which is a diuretic, but any treatment for blood pressure can cause postural hypotension and lead to falls

When you visit Mrs Gibson at home, you find she is on her own as both her son and daughter-in-law are at work. She denies falling but thinks she may have knocked herself on the furniture.

What general questions do you need to ask her?

- How she managing generally?
- Has she had any faints or 'funny turns'?
- Any major health worries or concerns?
- Has she lost any weight recently?
- Any indigestion or vomiting?
- Any trouble with her bowels or urinary symptoms? (Urinary tract infections are common in the elderly, particularly women)
- Is she taking any over-the-counter medications such as aspirin or 'flu or cold remedies'? These often contain aspirin and/or antihistamines.

Mrs Gibson says she is managing fine and denies any health problems apart from the ulcer on her leg. However, on examination she is very thin and has some large superficial dark bruises on both forearms and a laceration over her left eyebrow with a slight bump as well. She also has palmar erythema. Her left shin is covered with a dressing and her right leg reveals some varicose eczema but no ulceration.

What other physical examinations do you want to perform?

- Pulse rate and rhythm to exclude any arrhythmia
- Blood pressure sitting and standing to see if there is a postural drop
- Heart position and sounds
- Check for signs of heart failure: peripheral oedema, raised jugular venous pressure, late inspiratory crackles in the lung bases and wheeze because of her history of asthma. If you have a peak flow meter in your bag you could ask her to blow into it
- Abdominal examination for any enlarged organs

- Neurological assessment of muscle tone, strength, peripheral reflexes, sensation and proprioception to exclude a peripheral neuropathy

What features of the bruising might make you suspicious that this could be physical abuse rather than accidental?

As with child abuse cases, bilateral fingertip bruising on the arms from being roughly handled or any evidence of slapping such as a handprint. You should also ask Mrs Gibson herself if anyone has pushed her recently or been verbally abusive.

Mrs Gibson has some fading dark brown bruises on her forearms and a darker patch on one hand. There are no marks on her upper arms or evidence of having been mishandled. She has a few spider naevi on her chest and neck.

- *Pulse = 80 beats/min regular*
- *BP 150/80 mm Hg sitting and 130/82 mm Hg standing*
- *Peak flow = 320 L/min*

  Her breath sounds are normal and no wheeze is present. Abdominal examination is normal with no palpable liver. Mrs Gibson appears to have normal strength in her legs, can detect light touch and has normal proprioception in her toes. Ankle reflexes are absent. Plantar reflexes are normal as are knee jerks. There is no evidence of tremor.

  Mrs Gibson denies any physical or verbal abuse, but she is unable to recall how she got the bruises on her arms.

What is the significance of absent ankle reflexes?

According to Dick (2003), absent ankle reflexes may not be significant in the elderly as about 6% of over-65-year-olds will not demonstrate them (National Framework for Older People). It also depends how skilled the examiner is at eliciting them.

As Mrs Gibson seems a bit vague about how she got the bruises, you decide to do an abbreviated mental test for the elderly.

1 Age
2 Time
3 Remember an address: '43 North St, Manchester'
4 Year
5 'Where are we now?'
6 'Do you know who I am?'
7 Date of birth
8 Year of First World War

9 Name of present Prime Minister
10 Count backwards from 20 to 1

Mrs Gibson is orientated in time and space but cannot tell you the name of the Prime Minister or how old she is, although she knows her date of birth ('I'm getting on a bit now . . . I think I must be 70 or so.'). Her overall score is 7, whereas a normal score is 8 or more.

You notice a bottle of sherry in the corner of the room and decide to ask her how much she is drinking. Mrs Gibson says she has one or two glasses of sherry in the evening to help her sleep.

What investigations might you want to do on this home visit and why?

- Liver function tests including gamma glutamyl transferase (GGT) because the spider naevi and palmar erythema raise the possiblility of excessive alcohol and/or liver disease which might be contributing to easy bruising (Box 36)
- Clotting studies
- Full blood count and platelets to check for anaemia and/or thrombocytopenia
- Urea and electrolytes because she is taking a diuretic for her blood pressure
- Thyroid function tests – hypothyroidism is often insidious and can be associated with bruising. Hyperthyroidism can cause weight loss

---

Box 36 Palmar erythema and spider naevi

- *Palmar erythema* (reddening of the thenar and hypothenar eminences) may be a sign of chronic liver disease but may also be a normal finding
- *Spider naevi* are small angiomas which appear on the surface of the skin on the upper part of the body. They may be caused by liver disease (increased circulating oestrogen) or a normal finding. Large number of them are more suspicious of an underlying pathology

---

What are you going to say to Mrs Gibson about the blood tests and what will you do next?

You need to explain to her that you would like to do some blood tests which will help you find out why she is bruising easily and check her general health. You can reassure her that you have not found anything seriously wrong on examining her, but you are concerned that she has these marks on her forearms and is not sure how they occurred. You say you will be in touch in the next week to arrange a follow-up visit.

| *Mrs Gibson thanks you for coming to see her and says she is just going to pop out to the shops now.*

What else should you do?
It would be sensible to talk to Mrs Gibson's relatives to find out their views and also try to gather what sort of relationship they have with her. What questions would be useful?
- Any ideas about how the bruising occurred?
- Do you have any concerns about her health?
- Have you noticed any change in her memory recently?
- Is she eating and looking after herself adequately?
- Are there times when it is a big strain having her living with you?
- Have you ever worried about how much she is drinking?
- Do you have any plans for the future regarding her care?

A few days later the blood test results arrive at the surgery.

What do these results tell you and are there any other investigations you should do?
See Table 7.

Table 7 Results of Mrs Gibson's blood tests. Liver function tests, clotting studies and thyroid function tests are normal.

	Mrs Gibson's results	Normal ranges
GGT	89 IU/L	5–50 IU/L
Hb	11.5 g/dL	11.5–16.0 g/dL
MCV	104 fl	78–100 fl
Platelet count	110×10^9/L	$150–400 \times 10^9$/L
Serum urea	17 mmol/L	2.1–8.0 mmol/L
Serum creatinine	143 µmol/L	70–100 µmol/L
Serum sodium	142 mmol/L	135–145 mmol/L
Serum potassium	3.8 mmol/L	3.5–5.0 mmol/L

GGT, gamma glutamyl transferase; Hb, haemoglobin; MCV, mean cell volume.

Each laboratory in the UK provides a normal or reference value for each test but these will vary between laboratories, depending on different brands of tests they may use from different manufacturers and how the results are interpreted.

The blood test results suggest mild renal impairment because of the raised urea and creatinine (very common in the elderly) and possible alcohol abuse as the GGT is raised but the liver itself does not seem to have been affected yet. She also has a macrocytosis, mild thrombocytopenia and a haemoglobin just within normal limits.

You need to check her serum ferritin, vitamin B_{12} and folate levels. You decide to ask the district nurse to do these blood tests when she next visits Mrs Gibson.

Follow-up 10 days later
You manage to phone Mrs Gibson's daughter-in-law and arrange to see her after morning surgery on Friday. You now have the results of the other blood tests:
- Ferritin level of 32 ng/L (normal 20–200 ng/L)
- Vitamin B_{12} of 250 ng/L (normal 160–900 ng/L)
- Serum folate of 2.1 mg/L (normal 4.0–18.0 mg/L)

When you visit again and talk to the daughter-in-law, you are relieved to find that she seems very concerned about Mrs Gibson. They appear to have a good relationship and you think abuse of any sort is highly unlikely. However, Mrs Gibson's alcohol consumption has been worrying both her son and daughter-in-law for several months. They know that she buys her own sherry at the local off-licence but are not sure how many bottles she is getting through in a week as she can be quite devious about disposing of the evidence. They have noticed that she often has a poor appetite and does not eat properly. The daughter-in-law is very aware that Mrs Gibson is on her own for most of the day and her only outing is once a week to the social club on a Saturday night.

What should you do next and are there any changes you should make to Mrs Gibson's prescribed medicines?
You need to talk to Mrs Gibson about the amount of alcohol she is drinking and point out the dangers to her of consuming too much in a non-judgemental way. You can use the evidence of the blood tests to warn her that she may damage her liver if she continues to drink. You should also point out the benefits of cutting down her

consumption. These include more money to spend on other things, less bruising and fewer falls and feeling more alert and healthy. You could ask her about her interests and whether she might want to go to a day centre or other activity locally.

In the short term, you may want to try and reduce the 5 mg prednisolone, which will be contributing to making her skin thin (and has other side-effects such as increasing blood pressure, causing gastric irritation and ulceration). You do not want to exacerbate her asthma so you should arrange to monitor this closely by regular peak flow readings (the district nurse could help with this). You should also prescribe 5 mg/day folic acid as her serum folate was low and arrange to repeat the blood tests in a month.

You could also talk to the district nurse about day centres or places that might interest Mrs Gibson (e.g. bridge club, tea dances, t'ai chi) and get her out of the house and into a safe environment. Many elderly people drink because they are bored and lonely so tackling her social isolation may be very relevant.

Outcome. Mrs Gibson is not keen to go to any clubs or day centres, which she says will be 'full of oldies' who she does not know. She takes the folic acid intermittently and continues to drink more than is advisable. Her blood count and GGT levels remain much the same, despite your advice. Her leg ulcer continues to be a problem and she sometimes requires a course of antibiotics for the cellulitis that develops in that area.

You reduce the prednisolone to 2.5 mg for 2 weeks and monitor her peak flow readings which do not change substantially. However, soon after stopping the prednisolone completely, Mrs Gibson has a severe asthma attack and is admitted to hospital. She is discharged on oral steroids (40 mg/day prednislone) and it is suggested that she stays on a maintenance dose of 2.5 mg prednisolone to prevent further attacks. Her blood pressure rises a little to 160/100 mmHg and you are not sure if this is secondary to the steroids or to alcohol, or both.

As the GP, all you can do is ask her to come to the surgery or do a home visit, perhaps every 2 months, to keep an eye on her, examine her chest and blood pressure and carry out regular blood tests (urea and electrolytes, full blood count, liver function) to make sure her health is not deteriorating. It is also important to stay in touch with her son and daughter-in-law and be available to discuss their concerns.

CASE REVIEW

Mrs Gibson's case presents a challenge for the GP as she is not likely to change her behaviour substantially and her drinking is likely to lead to a deterioration in her health. Many people who drink excessively become malnourished because they get most of their calorie intake from the alcohol. They may not feel hungry and the alcohol itself may lead to gastritis and malabsorption, which in turn can lead to protein and vitamin deficiencies. Mrs Gibson is already folate deficient which can be treated with tablets. She is less in danger of becoming severely malnourished because she lives with her son and daughter-in-law who cook for her.

Any bruising that appears without a good reason needs further investigation. While it is common in the elderly to develop petechiae and ecchymoses because of skin thinning, physical abuse should be considered. It is difficult to raise this issue with the family and you need to get to know the circumstances and family dynamics in each individual case. Establishing a good relationship with Mrs Gibson's son and daughter-in-law and arranging regular reviews of her physical and mental state is very important in maintaining her current (fragile) health.

Interpreting blood test results in the elderly should be done with care and caution as renal function diminishes with age and thrombocytopenia is a common finding without necessarily being pathological in the absence of other blood abnormalities. If in doubt, it is sensible to get advice from a local pathologist or haematologist about whether further investigations are indicated.

Finally, alcohol misuse contributes to the problems of falls, depression, memory loss, osteoporosis and stroke. Alcohol also lowers the immune system and may make Mrs Gibson more vulnerable to chest and skin infections. While not wanting to take away one of Mrs Gibson's few pleasures, you should try and point out the benefits to her health of drinking less and encourage her to take up other activities instead.

KEY POINTS

- Bruising in the elderly is common and physical abuse must be considered as well as more common causes such as skin thinning and thrombocytopenia
- Oral steroids taken over long periods can lead to skin thinning
- Macrocytosis without anaemia is most likely to be caused by excess alcohol intake
- Alcohol interferes with folic acid absorption so folate deficiency is common in people with a poor diet and those who drink too much alcohol
- Many elderly people are lonely and socially isolated. Tackling this problem can be as important as sorting out their medical concerns
- 17% of men and 7% of older women drink more than the recommended limits
- Prescribing for the elderly should be done with care and reviewed regularly as renal function is often impaired
- Safe limits of alcohol for a woman = 14 units/week (1 unit = one small sherry of 90 mL or one glass of wine = 125 mL)

References

Dick, J.P. (2003) The deep tendon and abdominal reflexes. *Journal of Neurology, Neurosurgery and Psychiatry* **74**, 150–153.

National Service Framework for Older People. http://www.dh.gov.uk Accessed on 26 July 2007.

Case 18 A 38-year-old man with high blood pressure

This West Indian patient is new to the surgery and there are no summarized notes. He comes in to see you and tells you that he has high blood pressure (BP) and that he feels as if there is warmth in his head and he is tired and sluggish. He has a friend who is a doctor in London and he hands you a scrap of paper with amiloride written on it and he says this is what he wants.

What do you want to know?
- How does he know he has high BP?
- How long has he had it for?
- Assess to see if he is truly symptomatic
- Consider the secondary causes for hypertension, in view of the patient's age
- Assess his overall cardiovascular disease risk

He says he has had high blood pressure for 'some time' and he has had medications for it in the past but did not continue them because 'they did not work'. He denies headache, blurred vision, postural symptoms, chest pains, shortness of breath, faints or flushing. He says he has been generally tired and sluggish for many months, but he finds it difficult to be specific.

Assessment of cardiovascular disease risk

Assessing cardiovascular disease (CVD) risk is essential in terms of complete assessment of the patient and their cardiovascular system. The aim is to prevent CVD, angina, myocardial infarction, peripheral vascular disease and stroke. The assessment of risk is at best an estimate and this is an area of much research. The aim is to treat the cardiovascular system as a whole, all modifiable factors should be included, as treating one in isolation will be of limited benefit in the long term. The Joint British Societies (2005) point out that coexistent risk factors tend to have a multiplicative effect on CVD, therefore all risk factors should be assessed.

- *Low risk* <10% risk over 10 years of cardiovascular disease
- *Moderate risk* 10–20% risk over 10 years of cardiovascular disease
- *High risk* >20% risk over 10 years of cardiovascular disease

In the context of low overall CVD risk, a single raised modifiable risk factor may not need treatment (e.g. BP), unless it reaches a certain level (Fig. 7).

What further information is required to assess cardiovascular risk?
- Current smoking status
- Ever smoked
- Height
- Weight
- Ethnicity
- Family history of cardiovascular disease
- Medications
- Blood pressure
- Cardiovascular examination

He tells you that he has never smoked and both his parents died aged 71 of a stroke. When you measure his height and weight, he has a body mass index (BMI) of 28 (Box 37).

On this occasion his blood pressure is 162/95 mmHg, having measured it in both arms and taken an average of two readings.

Cardiovascular examination reveals pulse 92 beats/min, regular rhythm, normal heart sounds, no murmurs or bruits.

Box 37 Body mass index (BMI) calculator

$$BMI = \frac{weight\ (in\ kg)}{height\ (m)^2}$$

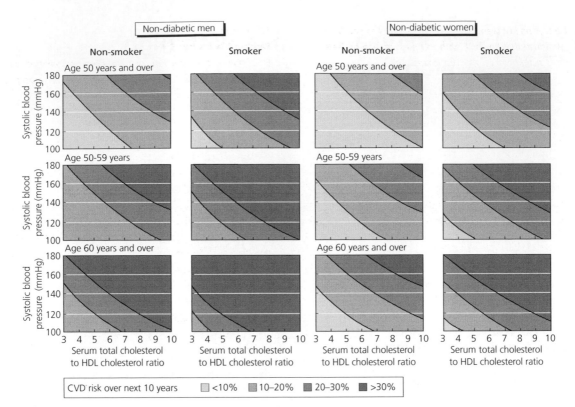

Figure 7 Cardiovascular disease (CVD) risk prediction charts. HDL, high density lipoprotein. From Beevers *et al.* (2007) *ABC of Hypertension*, 5th edn. Blackwells/BMJ with permission.

What should you tell him?

You should inform him that indeed his blood pressure is raised and you require further information to treat him appropriately. You should also say that you need to examine him further, and you require two further BP readings on different occasions (Box 38). Blood and urine tests to assess his cholesterol, kidney and liver function are needed.

What initial investigations would you carry out?

- Random glucose
- Renal function
- Liver function
- Lipids: total cholesterol and high density lipoprotein (HDL) cholesterol
- Urine dipstick for protein and sugar
- Fundoscopy
- ECG

Box 38 Measuring blood pressure

Most practices use digital BP devices. These are easy to use, but can be inaccurate if the pulse is irregular and can be uncomfortable (Prodigy Guidance).

Using a standard sphygmomanometer
- The cuff must be 40% of the arm circumference
- The bladder must be positioned over the brachial artery with the arm supported, in a temperate climate and the person quiet
- Palpate the artery while the cuff inflates, giving estimate of systolic BP. Inflate to 30 mmHg above systolic pressure and deflate at 2 mmHg/s
- Measure both arms, usually using the higher reading. Use an average of two readings

He says he just wants this tablet (amiloride) as you have confirmed that he has high blood pressure and he feels there is no need for any further tests.

It is important not to underestimate patient's ideas and expectations. Health beliefs can be strongly held, as they may have a family or cultural origin and have been engrained over the patient's lifetime (Williams 2006).

How should you respond?

You confirm that you have understood his concerns and are taking on board his requests but you discuss the need to do your very best for him and that requires further information in the form of blood tests and urine investigations.

He agrees to see the practice nurse for a BP check and these investigations and you see him again in 2 weeks.

You give him a leaflet regarding lifestyle interventions for reducing cardiovascular risk: exercise, salt intake, healthy diet, weight reduction. This may seem to devalue the importance of modification of lifestyle factors, but this just plants the seed. At another occasion, when he may be more receptive, they can be tackled in depth.

What would you do next?
In 2 weeks

- Record another BP reading
- Estimate CVD risk (Box 39)
- Look at ECG and blood tests
- Discuss treatment if necessary and a way to pitch a different medicine other than the one that he wants
- Discuss modification of lifestyle factors

Box 39 Tools for the estimation of cardiovascular risk

- Tables in the back of the *BNF* (based on Framingham studies)
- On-line calculators
- Calculators on GP computer systems

Results

BP readings with practice nurse, 164/96 and 163/92 mmHg

U&E, Na 142, K 4.5, Ur 6.2, Cr 97

Total cholesterol (TC) 6.2

HDL cholesterol 0.8

TC : HDL ratio 7.7

Random blood sugar 5.7

ECG, normal sinus rhythm, rate 84, does not meet voltage criteria for left ventricular hypertrophy (LVH), no ischaemic changes

10-year CVD risk – 12%

Does this confirm whether he needs any treatment?

On the basis of the information above, this man requires treatment for his BP as he has three readings persistently over 160/90 mmHg (Box 40). His overall CVD risk (12.2%) does not mean he needs treatment for his lipids and he does not require aspirin prophylaxis. A cardiovascular risk of 20% or more would require treatment for lipids also. It would be prudent, however, to discuss dictary modifications to reduce his weight and improve his lipid profile.

Box 40 Thresholds and targets

NICE (2006). Hypertension is persistent raised blood pressure: on at least two visits, systolic or diastolic pressure or both are above 140/90 mmHg.

Offer treatment if BP 160/100 mmHg or isolated hypertension >160 mmHg or BP >140/90 mmHg and 10-year cardiovascular risk >20% or existing CVD or target organ damage. Aim to reduce BP to 140/90 mmHg or below.

How do you convey risk, how is this useful?

Compared with men who do not have hypertension (who would have a 10-year CVD risk of 8–9%), he has approximately 50% greater chance of developing heart disease or stroke. His 12% risk means, out of eight men who are the same, one of those over the next 10 years will develop heart disease or stroke.

In this case you do not have to convince him that treatment should be seriously considered, rather which treatment he should choose.

Having explained all of the information to him, you tell him that treatment for his blood pressure is recommended. You ask why, in particular, he asks for this medicine, and he says that his friend in London, who is a heart doctor, recommended this to him. He feels that this friend is at the top of his game and trusts him.

You inform him that you do not feel amiloride is a good first choice antihypertensive medication because it is principally used to treat swelling of the legs (oedema) and only used for certain people with high blood pressure (i.e. in hypertension treatment if hypokalaemia develops; *BNF* 2.2.4 Potassium-sparing diuretics). You ask him if he would be open to other suggestions for treatment that are better at bringing down blood pressure and tell him that they are also recommended by experts. He agrees and you discuss with him the following options (Fig. 8).

As he is a West Indian man, the treatment options include calcium channel blockers (Box 41) and thiazide diuretics (Box 42).

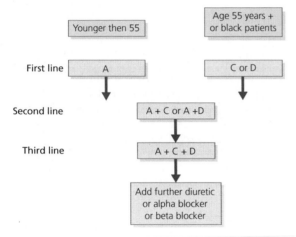

Figure 8 Treatment of newly diagnosed hypertension. β-blockers are not used except for patients with acute myocardial infarction/ angina/congestive cardiac failure. A, angiotensin converting enzyme (ACE) inhibitor (consider angiotensin II receptor antagonist if ACE intolerant); C, calcium channel blocker; D, thiazide-type diuretic. From NICE (2006).

> **Box 41 Calcium channel blockers (e.g. felodipine)**
>
> - *Efficacy and safety:* similar (Staessen *et al.* 2001)
> - *Starting dose:* 5 mg o.d.
> - *Side-effects:* flushing, headache palpitations, dizziness, fatigue, oedema (for full side-effect profile see *BNF* 54, 2.6.2, p. 112)

> **Box 42 Thiazide diuretics (e.g. bendromethiazide)**
>
> - Efficacy and safety: similar (Staessen *et al.* 2001)
> - *Dose:* 2.5 mg o.d.
> - *Side-effects:* include postural hypotension, gastrointestinal disturbance, impotence, biochemical disturbance (for full side-effect profile see *BNF* 54, 2.2.1, p. 72)

He opts for a calcium channel blocker, felodipine. He agrees that the side-effects sound less when compared with thiazide diuretics. You discuss the medication, how to take it and emphasize that the treatment generally will be lifelong. You arrange to see him for follow-up in 4 weeks time.

> **KEY POINTS**
>
> - Understand and address the problem from the patient's perspective (e.g. belief about causation of symptoms and treatment options)
> - Identify hypertension by measuring blood pressure over three occasions
> - 40% of the adult population have sustained high BP >140/90 mmHg
> - Hypertension increases with age, and has a higher prevalence in Afro-Caribbean men and women and in South Asians
> - Offer lifestyle advice initially and then periodically to patients undergoing assessment or treatment
> - In patients with no established CVD, assess cardiovascular risk
> - Careful and comprehensive cardiovascular risk assessment
> - Be prepared to discuss the meaning of risk
> - Consider the need for specialist investigation of patients with signs and symptoms suggesting a secondary cause of hypertension
> - Offer drug therapy if persistent BP 160/100 mmHg or patients with BP 140/90 mmHg and raised CVD risk

References

Beevers, G., Lip, G. & O'Brien, E., (eds.) (2007) *ABC of Hypertension*, 5th edn. Blackwell/BMJ Books, Oxford.

PART 2: CASES

British National Formulary 54 (2007) BMJ Publishing and RPS Publishing, London.

Joint British Societies. (2005) Guidelines on the prevention of cardiovascular disease in clinical practice. *Heart* **91** (Suppl v), v1–v52.

National Institute for Health and Clinical Excellence (NICE). (2006) *Hypertension: Management of Hypertension in Adults in Primary Care.* Clinical guideline No. 34. NICE, London.

Prodigy guidance. *Hypertension.* http://cks.library.nhs.uk/hypertension/in_depth/background_information Accessed on 7 May 2007.

Staessen, J.A., Wang, J-G. & Thijs, L. (2001) Cardiovascular protection and blood pressure reduction; a meta-analysis. *Lancet* **358**, 1305–1315.

Williams, L.A.D. (2006) Ethnomedicine. *West Indian Medical Journal* **55** (4). caribbean.scielo.org/scielo.php?script=sci_arttext&pid=S0043-31442006000400001&lng=pt&nrm=iso&tlng=en Accessed on 2 May 2007.

Case 19 An 80-year-old woman with funny turns

You are diligently attending to paperwork prior to surgery one morning. You notice that one of your 'book on the day' slots has just been given out and the lady, Miss Ivy Brown has already arrived.

Your inquisitive nature takes hold and you check her records. She is 80, lives alone and has not been in contact with the surgery since 2005. Last winter she refused her flu vaccine and is on no regular medications. You note she has no home phone number, but there is the name of her friend on the screen with a contact telephone number.

After deciding to have an extra few minutes in the consultation you call her in. She appears a bit pale and sits down heavily. 'Now then,' you say, 'You are up early. What can I do for you?'

'Well,' she says, 'I don't like to bother you for something so trivial but it just won't go away.' You enquire further. She says she is having trouble doing her usual chores because of her 'funny dos', and she just cannot shake them off.

What are the possible differential diagnoses?

This is a very common situation in primary care, where the presenting complaint, 'funny dos' does not fit neatly into any one clear category (Jones *et al.* 2003, section 1.3). Therefore, the list of differential diagnoses is unfortunately long and sometimes it is difficult to narrow it down. It may be useful to enlist the help of a witness to give a description of what she or he observes at the time of a 'funny do'.

- Cardiovascular
  - Arrythmias
  - Syncope
  - Postural hypotension
- Neurological
  - Transient ischaemic attack (TIA)/stroke
  - Multiple sclerosis
  - Epilepsy

- ENT
  - Labyrinthine disorders
  - Benign positional vertigo
  - Ménière's disease
- Haematological
  - Anaemia
- Metabolic
  - Hypoglycaemia
  - Thyroid disease
- Psychological
  - Anxiety
  - Depression

What further questions would you like to ask?

- What do you mean by 'funny do's'?
- How long have they been going on for?
- How long do they last?
- Is there anything else you have noticed when you are having a funny do such as feeling sick, feeling breathless or needing to go to the toilet?
- What brings them on?
- What makes them worse?
- Have you had any falls?
- Do you ever black out or lose conciousness?
- Have you had any similar episodes in the past?

Miss Brown confirms they have been going on for 3–4 months and describes her 'funny do's' by saying it feels like she must sit down, and her head is a little fuzzy and she cannot do the hoovering. She says there is no vertigo or room spinning. She occasionally feels faint and she says she has fallen four times, but is not sure if she has blacked out. The episodes last for 15–20 min and they go off of their own accord.

You ask specifically if she notices any strange feelings before she feels faint (aura, hallucination, chest pain, palpitations, shortness of breath, nausea, sweating, disturbed vision).

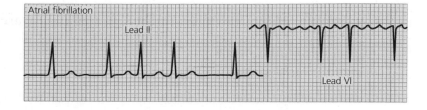

Figure 9 Electrocardiogram (ECG) showing atrial fibrillation with typical absence of P waves and irregular QRS complexes.

She tells you she occasionally has palpitations, which can precede feeling faint, with no chest pain, nausea or sweating. She says that the palpitations are a feeling that her heart is beating very fast indeed.

Differential diagnosis of palpitations?

Longmore *et al.* (2002) and gpnotebook.co.uk

Intrinsic causes

- Arrythmias
    - Supraventricular tachycardia (SVT) – atrial fibrillation or atrial flutter
    - Heart block
    - Atrial or ventricular ectopics
- Syncope
- Valvular disorders

Extrinsic causes

- Drugs; caffeine, cocaine, β-blockers, alcohol
- Metabolic; thyroid disorders
- Exercise
- Anxiety

What should you do next?

Examine of the cardiovascular system.

You ask Miss Brown if you may examine her and if she is experiencing any palpitations now, she replies yes to both.

On examination, she looks pale but not unduly short of breath and she is able to talk in complete sentences. Her pulse is irregularly irregular with a rate of 132 beats/min. Her BP is 100/80 mmHg with a manual blood pressure machine. Her apex rate is 152 beats/min, with no discernable murmurs. She has bilateral crackles in her lung bases.

What is the most appropriate course of action?

From the history, she is describing recurrent palpitations and the examination suggests fast atrial fibrillation (AF)

with evidence of haemodynamic compromise (low blood pressure) and heart failure (crackles in the lungs). An ECG is required to confirm the clinical suspicion of fast AF (Fig. 9). However, in view of these findings and her social situation you recommend acute medical assessment at the local hospital.

What are you going to say to Miss Brown?

We have found the reason why you are having funny do's and fainting. You heart is beating very fast and irregularly. It is too fast to keep up with the demands of your body. We know it is struggling because your blood pressure is low. It is important that this is treated now because of the strain on your heart and because AF increases the risk of stroke.

She initially refuses to be admitted as she feels she is not prepared for this and has not packed an overnight bag. She seems shocked and upset by this news as she hoped there was nothing wrong. You ask her if she would like us to contact her friend to inform her of the situation. You ask the practice nurse to talk things through with her and to contact her friend while you inform the admitting medical officer and ask reception to call for an ambulance.

Her friend is able to talk to her, and again impress on her the urgency of the situation, reassure her that she will meet her there and bring some belongings from her home.

Two days later she is discharged from hospital and comes to see you because she is unsure about her medication.

How should you respond?

You explain that AF or fast fluttering of the heart has been confirmed and unfortunately that puts her at an increased risk of a stroke (Box 43). You can reassure her by saying that this problem is common at her age and can be successfully controlled with medication.

Box 43 Atrial fibrillation

Longmore *et al.* (2002)
- Prevalence of 9% in those over 75 years of age
- Aetiological factors: ischaemic heart disease and myocardial infarction, heart failure, hypertension, mitral valve disease, pneumonia, hyperthyroidism and alcohol
- The main complication is embolic stroke

She tells you she is on digoxin and warfarin. She wants to know when she can stop them. She hands you a copy of the discharge summary from the hospital.

What are the therapeutic strategies?

There are two therapeutic strategies in the treatment of AF:

1 Rate control or rhythm control
2 Antithrombotic treatment

Miss Brown does fit into the rate control category (Box 44) and hence has been commenced on digoxin. The therapeutic options for rate control include digoxin, β-blockers and rate-limiting calcium antagonists. Digoxin is usually only used in those who are sedentary, mainly the elderly. This is because it has a poor effect in hyper-adrenergic states (in exercise, fever, thyrotoxiscosis; Shantsila *et al.* 2007).

Antiplatelet treatment or thromboprophylaxis is indicated in all cases to reduce the risk of stroke. Depending on the presence of other risk factors for stroke, anticoagulation with warfarin or antiplatelet treatment with aspirin should be recommended.

Name...... *Miss Ivy Brown*	Consultant......... *Dr Williams*
Address.... *64 ACRE LANE*	Speciality...... *Elderly*
LEEDS	Ward............ *56*
LS17 9NM	Admitted.......... *14/5/07*
	Discharge........ *17/5/07*
Date of Birth........... *19/7/28*	Address on Discharge...... *As over*

Clinical information..........

AF
ECG - AF
ECHO - Mild LVH, Impaired LV function
Digoxin started
Warfarin started

Discharge Medications

Drug	Dose	Frequency	Quantity	Pharmacy Check
DIGOXIN	*125 micrograms*	*OD*	*14*	
WARFARIN	*2mg*	*OD as per INR*	*14*	

Discharge Medications

Drugs started	Drugs stopped
DIGOXIN	
WARFARIN	

Follow-up arrangements

Anticoagulant Clinic 1 week

Doctor	Nurse	Pharmacist

PART 2: CASES

> **Box 44 NICE guidelines for the management of AF (2006) suggest rate control in the following circumstances**
>
> If the patient is:
> - Over 65 years
> - Has coronary heart disease
> - Has contraindications to antiarrythmic drugs
> - Is unsuitable for cardioversion

> **Box 45 Risk of bleeding**
>
> Consider bleeding risk carefully in those:
> - Over 75 years
> - Taking antiplatelet medication (e.g. aspirin and clopidogrel) and non-steroidal anti-inflammatory drugs
> - Taking multiple other drugs
> - With uncontrolled hypertension
> - With a history of bleeding (e.g. peptic ulcer or cerebral haemorrhage)
> - With a history of poorly controlled anticoagulation therapy

Who is at high risk of stroke?

NICE (2006):
- Previous TIA/stroke or thromboembolic event
- Age >75 years with hypertension, diabetes or vascular disease
- Clinical evidence of heart failure, or impaired left ventricular function on ECHO

Is Miss Brown at high risk of stroke?

In this given situation, Miss Brown fits into the high risk group, because of her left ventricular hypertrophy (LVH) and mildly impaired left ventricular function on ECHO. In these cases, warfarin is recommended unless contraindicated.

How would you explain this to the patient?

Treatment with warfarin should be discussed with the patient, in terms of risk and benefits. The stroke rate per year in the high risk group in the elderly is 8% without thromboprophylaxis, 4–5% per year on aspirin and 1–2% on warfarin (Jones *et al.* 2003).

Assessment of the patient's suitability for warfarin

Prior to the commencement of warfarin, a careful assessment is necessary including the risk of bleeding (Box 45), ability to understand instructions and risk of falling should be undertaken. In this case, Miss Brown does not have a home telephone, and this poses risks if there is an urgent need for medical attention. Following discussion with her and her friend she contacts BT to install a land line.

How to convey risk to patients?

The aim is to present information in a usable and understandable format to enable patients to make informed choices about their own health and treatment. To individualize risk estimates, in multiple formats (descrip-

Table 8 Stroke rate in high risk group (Jones *et al.* 2003).

Thromboprophylaxis option	No treatment	Aspirin	Warfarin
Stroke rate per year (%)	8	4–5	1–2

tively and numerically) have been reported to be the most effective approach (Table 8; Jones *et al.* 2003).

Descriptive framing

In this given situation with Miss Brown, she is at high risk of stoke. If aspirin is started, she is less likely to have a stroke, and if she takes warfarin she is even less likely to have a stroke.

Numerical framing

Miss Brown has a 1 in 12 annual risk of stroke. The risk is reduced by 50% if aspirin is taken. If warfarin is taken this risk is reduced further by 75% (relative risk reduction).

What information should you give to Miss Brown who is taking warfarin?

Warfarin is used to reduce the risk of stroke. It works by making the blood less sticky. It can reduce your risk of stroke by up to half. There is a concern with warfarin, that because the blood is less sticky bleeding is more likely following an injury. Blood testing is necessary for monitoring that will initially be frequently, every week, and when the dose is stable, up to every 3 months. The blood tests are called international normalized ratio (INR) and are usually carried out at the local anticoagulation clinic, here at the surgery or at the hospital. You will be given your own personal record book which has results, dosing instructions and the date of the next test. The dose taken may change depending upon blood test results.

Care must be exercised when taking other medications (including antibiotics and over-the-counter remedies, especially St John's Wort), and when making significant changes to your diet (including salad and vegetables) and the amount of alcohol you drink. This is because any significant change can alter the metabolism of warfarin and therefore the INR (*BNF 54* 2007, Interactions).

You must tell all doctors or nurses that you are on warfarin, particularly if you are admitted to hospital or they change your medicines.

Outcome. Miss Brown decided to continue with her warfarin and digoxin treatments. She did feel the visits for blood tests were inconvenient but she persevered. She now resides in a nursing home following a further admission to hospital with a stroke. She is unfortunately struggling with depression after her stroke and the loss of her independence.

CASE REVIEW

- Miss Browns' presentation was out of character and should heighten the suspicion to a genuine problem
- Careful history taking takes a broad and non-specific symptom (funny turns) and funnels towards a workable differential diagnosis (palpitations)
- In this case, examination confirmed the diagnosis
- Involving Miss Brown in all steps of the management was important as compliance with investigations and treatment was essential
- Assessment of individual risk for stroke and bleeding was carried out for Miss Brown, and treatment was tailored accordingly
- Reassessment of risk should be undertaken regularly

KEY POINTS

- 'Funny do's' are a common and difficult presentation
- Treatable, life-threatening causes should be considered
- Atrial fibrillation is common, with a prevalence of 9% in those over 75 years
- Atrial fibrillation is the most common arrhythmia and contributes to 15% of all strokes (Shantsila *et al.* 2007)
- Atrial fibrillation is increasingly common with age, hypertension, heart failure, coronary artery disease and diabetes mellitus (Longmore *et al.* 2002)
- Primary care investigations include initial blood tests and ECG
- Informed choice is of great importance to ensure compliance with treatments, especially medications

References

British National Formulary 54. (2007) British Medical Society and Royal Pharmaceutical Society of Great Britain, London.

GP Notebook. www.gpnotebook.co.uk Accessed on 7 December 2007.

Jones, R., Britten, N., Culpepper, L., Gass, D.A., Grol, R., Mant, D., *et al.* (2003) *Oxford Textbook of Primary Medical Care*. Oxford University Press, Oxford.

Longmore, M., Wilkinson, I. & Torok, E. (2002) *Oxford Handbook of Clinical Medicine*, 5th edn. Oxford University Press, Oxford.

National Institute of Health and Clinical Excellence (NICE). (2006) *Atrial Fibrillation. The management of atrial fibrillation*. Clinical guideline No. 36. NICE, London.

Shantsila, E., Watson, T. & Lip, G. (2007) Current management of atrial fibrillation in older people. *Prescriber* **18**, 49–53.

Case 20   A 43-year-old man with 'weakness'

Mr Khan, a patient originally from Pakistan, comes to see you and says he is feeling 'weak'. He is not able to elaborate but it seems to have been going on for several months. You notice he looks rather grey and you can smell nicotine when he walks into the room. He is wrapped up in several layers of clothing on top of his tunic and trousers and is wearing a woollen hat. You remember that he is the proud father of five children, including Mohammed, a 2-year-old with eczema (see Case 12).

Feeling 'weak' is a common but non-specific presentation in general practice. What else should you ask him?

- Is he sleeping all right?
- Any other symptoms such as breathlessness or pain anywhere (could this be anaemia, malignancy or heart disease)?
- How is his appetite and general health?
- What did he think might be wrong?

You are aware that Mr Khan works night shifts as a taxi driver and generally tries to sleep in the day so this might be contributing to the problem.

Mr Khan says he is sleeping reasonably, although the children often disturb him, but he does not wake up feeling refreshed. He has not noticed any other symptoms and is not breathless. His appetite has been fine but general health 'not good'. He is not sure what might be wrong but his older brother was diagnosed with diabetes last year and he wants to be checked for this.

What other questions might you ask him, given this information about the family history of diabetes?

- Has he been more thirsty recently?
- Has he been passing more urine than usual?
- Has he had any recent infections (bacterial and fungal skin infections are more common in people with a raised blood sugar)?
- Has he noticed any change in his vision (this is particularly relevant as he is a taxi driver)?

Mr Khan says he has been thirsty and drinking more, but has not had any of the other symptoms.

What should you do next?

A general examination is a good idea to look for signs of anaemia, measure his blood pressure and listen to his heart and lungs, particularly as he is a smoker. You should record his weight and height and ask him for a sample of urine.

It takes a few minutes for him to remove his layers of clothes.

Findings:
No obvious anaemia on inspection of nails and conjunctivae
Pulse 76 beats/min, regular
BP 136/74 mmHg
Heart sounds normal, chest clear and abdominal examination normal apart from excess weight
Body mass index (BMI) 28.9 (weight 87.4 kg, height 174 cm) BMI >25.0 is overweight
Waist circumference 105 cm (ideal is <90 cm)
Urinalysis: glucose +++, protein+, ketones, nitrites, leucocytes and blood – negative
Finger prick blood test – glucometer gives a blood sugar of 17 mmol/L

What are you going to say to Mr Khan?

You tell him that his suspicions were right and that he does have a raised blood sugar, suggesting a diagnosis of diabetes. This condition greatly increases his risk of cardiovascular disease, but so also does his smoking and increased weight. (Both his BMI and large waist circumference confirm this.) You follow this up by emphasizing that Mr Khan can do much himself to control the diabetes, prevent the disease getting worse and lower his risks of developing heart and circulation problems. You are also aware that type 2 diabetes is much more common in the South Asian population in the UK and carries a higher risk of heart and kidney disease than among the European population.

What should you ask him now?

Prodigy guidance (2007):

• What does he know already about diabetes?

• How much does he smoke?

• Does he drink any alcohol (most has a high sugar content)?

• Does he do any regular exercise?

• Is there anyone else in the family with diabetes and/or heart disease?

> *Mr Khan is quite philosophical about the diagnosis as his brother seems to cope well and is just on tablets. He knows that diabetes is a serious condition and can lead to problems if the blood sugar is too high, although he is quite vague about what these problems are. He smokes 10–15 cigarettes a day and does not drink alcohol. He takes no regular exercise.*
>
> *There is a strong family history of diabetes as both his parents have it, as well as two of his older brothers. His father back in Pakistan, now aged 66, had an heart attack in his late fifties and is on treatment for angina. His mother also has high blood pressure.*

You glance at your watch and realize you are running 15 min late and you can hear a crying baby in the waiting room. You decide to arrange to see Mr Khan again soon for a longer appointment to explain more fully about the diagnosis of diabetes. You give him two patient information leaflets, one in his own language, Urdu, and one in English (www.patient.co.uk) about diabetes, as well as a diet sheet about healthy eating and avoidance of sugar.

What investigations should you organize now before you see him again in a few days?

• Fasting blood glucose to confirm the diagnosis

• Glycosylated haemoglobin (HbA1c)

• Fasting lipids

• Urea and electrolytes for kidney function

• Liver function tests

As there are no ketones in the urine and this is not an emergency situation, you ask Mr Khan to make an appointment with the practice nurse as soon as possible and to starve for 12 h before the blood tests. You arrange a double appointment to see you again 5 days after this.

Mr Khan wants to know whether he can go to work tonight?

It is likely that Mr Khan has had diabetes for some time and his blood sugar is not dangerously high. As he has no neurological symptoms and has not noticed any sig-

nificant changes in his vision, he is able to drive. You are not quite sure about the Driving Vehicle Licensing Agency (DVLA) rules on diabetes and say you will check this before you see him again. You ask Mr Khan to avoid eating all sugar at the moment and to read the information leaflets so he can come prepared to ask you some more questions at the next appointment.

When a patient develops type 2 diabetes, the issues that need to be discussed are complex and many. It can feel overwhelming for both the health professional and the patient to try and tackle all of these at one time. The patient will not remember everything and you will not have time to cover all aspects. You decide that when you see Mr Khan again, you will concentrate on three topics:

1 Blood test results

2 Diet

3 Smoking

Your main task is educating Mr Khan about diabetes, arranging appropriate referrals for retinal screening and to a dietitian, and helping him to lower his risk factors for developing complications of the disease in the long term. Key people who can help with this educational and support process are the practice nurse, the local hospital (which may run educational sessions for people with newly diagnosed diabetes) and voluntary organizations such as Diabetes UK (www.diabetes.org.uk). In some areas, there may be a specialist diabetic nurse who will see patients at home with their family.

The following week

Mr Khan's blood results are as follow.

> *Fasting blood sugar 10.3 mmol/L*
> *HbA1c 9.7% (<7.0%)*
> *Total cholesterol 6.4 mmol/L (<4.0 mmol/L)*
> *High density lipoprotein (HDL-C) 3.9 mmol/L (>1.0 mmol/L)*
> *Low density lipoprotein (LDL-C) 2.7 mmol/L (<2.5 mmol/L)*
> *Triglycerides 1.9 mmol/L (1.7 mmol/L)*
> *Urea and electrolytes – normal*
> *Full blood count – normal*
> *Liver function tests – normal*

Diabetes can be diagnosed on the basis of one abnormal plasma glucose (random >11.0 mmol/L or fasting blood sugar >7.0 mmol/L) in the presence of diabetic symptoms such as thirst or increased urination. As Mr Khan has noticed that he has been more thirsty recently, a second test is not required.

The glycosylated haemoglobin level reflects the average blood glucose over the last 3 months. The aim is to keep it below 7% to lower the risk of complications from diabetes and achieve good blood sugar control.

You check the DVLA website (www.dvla.gov.uk) and find that Mr Khan does not need to inform them about the diabetes if he is not on treatment and his visual acuity is satisfactory, that is 6/6 in at least one eye. You make a note in his records that this will need checking again when his blood sugar is controlled.

Mr Khan arrives for his appointment. He looks tired and depressed. When you ask him how he is feeling, he shakes his head and says he is 'not good'. You explain what you are going to cover in this consultation and what might need leaving for another time (such as exercise and medication). Finally, you would like to give him the chance to ask any questions he has.

What do you say about the blood tests?

You explain that the tests confirm that he does have type 2 diabetes, a raised HbA1c level and slightly higher than ideal fats in his blood. However, all the other results are normal. Blood sugar is controlled in the body by the hormone insulin which is produced in the pancreas. Some people develop diabetes when they are not producing enough insulin or when the body ceases to use insulin effectively. You say that the main problem with a raised blood sugar is that it can affect the blood vessels and cause damage to them, leading to circulation and heart problems and sometimes affecting the vision. These complications can be avoided if the blood sugar is kept under control and other risk factors are tackled, such as his smoking and diet.

Mr Khan says he just wants the tablets to treat his diabetes and then he will be fine.

You explain that at this stage, tablets are not indicated as he may well respond to diet alone. He should try this for at least 3 months before medication is considered. You offer to refer him to see a dietitian and suggest that his wife might want to go to the appointment as well. You ask him what his usual diet is like.

Mr Khan tells you that he eats rice and curry (meat or fish) most days with vegetables. He drinks tea with sugar and has a can of cola when he is out in the taxi. He does not have many sugary foods such as biscuits or cakes.

What is a good balanced diet for someone with diabetes (or anyone)?

• Reducing fat (especially saturated fat) in the diet
• Increasing fruit and vegetable consumption
• Increasing intake of fibre-rich starchy foods, such as bread and rice
• Reducing salt intake
• Increasing fish (especially oily fish) intake
• Decreasing sugar intake
• Diet based on energy intake (55–60% carbohydrate, 15–20% protein and 20–30% fat) improves diabetic control and lipid levels and helps to maintain body weight. The addition of dietary fibre also improves diabetic control and lipid levels (Prodigy guidance 2007)

You suggest to Mr Khan that he should use a synthetic sweetener in his tea and buy sugar-free cola or switch to an alternative low-calorie drink.

What about lowering his risk of cardiovascular disease with the use of statins?

You check the Joint British Societies Coronary Risk Prediction Chart (Joint British Societies Coronary Risk Prediction Chart in the back of the *BNF*) which works out the risk of a patient developing cardiovascular problems based on the ratio of the total serum cholesterol (TC) to the HDL cholesterol. In Mr Khan's case the TC : HDL ratio is 6.4/1–6 = 4.0. At this level and with a systolic blood pressure of 134 mmHg, looking at the table for smokers with diabetes, Mr Khan's coronary heart disease risk is less than 15% over the next 10 years, so statins are not indicated (NICE October 2002), although this is controversial. Some doctors are now recommending that statins should be prescribed for all those with type 2 diabetes because of the threefold increase in cardiovascular risk, particularly in high risk ethnic groups such as South Asians.

Should he be prescribed aspirin?

The Joint British Societies (2005) guideline on prevention of cardiovascular disease issued in 2005 recommends: 'Aspirin 75 mg daily is recommended for all people with type 2 diabetes who are 50 years of age, and selectively in younger people with one of the following criteria: (1) who have had the disease for more than 10 years; (2) or who are already receiving treatment for hypertension; (3) or who have evidence of target organ damage in the form of retinopathy or nephropathy, and whose blood pressure is controlled to at least <150/90 mmHg, and preferably to the optimal target of <130/80 mmHg.' According to these guidelines, it is premature to prescribe aspirin for Mr Khan at this stage.

Anyone with a diagnosis of type 2 diabetes should be screened annually for retinopathy so you explain to Mr Khan that you will be referring him to the hospital to have the back of his eyes examined, as this investigation can pick up any early changes in the blood vessels that might need treatment.

Your 20 min appointment with Mr Khan is nearly at an end. You decide to raise the issue of his smoking and ask him if he has ever considered stopping.

Mr Khan says he does not smoke a lot and although he knows it is not good for him, he has never tried to give up although his wife has urged him to in the past.

You point out some of the advantages of giving up smoking, including lowering his risks of heart disease and cancer and saving money. As he is the main breadwinner in the family and has five dependent children and a wife at home, looking after his own health is crucial. You tell him about the smoking cessation clinic at the practice which will provide information and support when he is ready to give up and ask him to discuss this further with the practice nurse.

Mr Khan still looks depressed and you ask him if he has any questions for you?

He says he is worried that he will lose his job as a taxi driver now that he has diabetes. He still thinks tablets would 'cure' him and is surprised that he is not being given any treatment.

You show Mr Khan the DVLA rules on diabetes and reassure him that there is no reason why he should not continue in his job as long as he has regular check-ups for his diabetes and in particular his eyesight. You explain again that taking tablets will not 'cure' the problem. He will end up having to take medication, but can delay this by altering his diet and improving his blood sugar control at this stage. You try to reassure him that with help from yourself and the practice nurse, he will soon understand how to manage the condition himself and feel better.

What follow-up should be arranged?

You can see that Mr Khan is not entirely happy or convinced about your management. You offer to see him and his wife at another appointment in 2 weeks. You also ask him to see the practice nurse to have his eyesight checked, discuss smoking cessation and exercise. He should bring a urine sample with him. You tell Mr Khan that he will be invited to attend the practice's diabetic clinic on a regular basis and that the nurse will tell him about the local education classes for newly diagnosed diabetics which are held at the hospital.

CASE REVIEW

The presentation of type 2 diabetes can vary and does not always fit the textbook description of a patient with polyuria, polydipsia and weight loss. It is not uncommon for people to complain of weakness or non-specific symptoms of feeling unwell. The key to good management is patient education and a team approach with other health professional colleagues in the community.

Mr Khan's case is complex because he has several risk factors for developing both microvascular (kidneys and eyes) and macrovascular (coronary arteries and arteries supplying the brain and feet) complications. Hopefully, with increased understanding of the condition, he will be motivated to make lifestyle changes that will lower these risks, particularly stopping smoking and modifying his diet. However, it is likely that he will end up taking tablets (probably metformin) to control his blood sugar.

You should offer to see his wife as well. This can be supportive for the patient and if she does most of the cooking it is very relevant to educate her about a healthy diet. You also know that their 2-year-old with eczema is overweight, which will increase his chances of developing diabetes in the future.

Lifestyle interventions and patient education should be individually tailored. In Mr Khan's case, as he is a shift worker, attention to when he is able to eat and what food is available may be relevant, particularly in the future if he has to start taking hypoglycaemic medication.

As type 2 diabetes is a progressive disease, there should be ongoing structured evaluation of cardiovascular and microvascular disease which will include:

- HbA1c measurements at 2–6 monthly intervals (NICE September 2002) with the aim to keep it at 6.5–7.5%
- Blood sugar monitoring
- Inspection of the feet (assessment of pulses and vibration sense)
- Blood pressure
- Urinanalyis for proteinuria and if present, subsequent testing for microalbuminuria to detect early kidney damage
- Medication review
- Assessment of visual acuity

KEY POINTS

- South Asians have a four- to fivefold increase in risk of developing type 2 diabetes compared to Europeans
- Diabetes tends to develop about 10 years earlier than in Europeans and complications such as kidney and heart disease are more common in South Asians
- South Asians have the highest death rates for coronary heart disease in the UK
- There is controversy over at what stage of the disease aspirin and statins should be prescribed
- With good control of blood sugar levels, the risk of complications of the disease can be minimized
- Interventions to control the disease should be individually tailored
- Patient education is crucial to improve understanding of the disease and to encourage responsibility for maintaining a healthy lifestyle
- A team approach to management of a patient with type 2 diabetes is important
- Doctors and patients need to be aware of the DVLA rules regarding diabetes and fitness to drive

References

British Cardiac Society; British Hypertension Society; Diabetes UK; HEART UK; Primary Care Cardiovascular Society; Stroke Association. (2005) JBS Joint British Societies' guidelines on prevention of cardiovascular disease in clinical practice. *Heart* **91** (Suppl 5), 1–52.

Diabetes UK – one of the largest charities in the UK. www.diabetes.org.uk

Driver Vehicle Licensing Agency (DVLA). *At a glance medical aspects of fitness to drive*. www.dvla.gov.uk

Joint British Societies Coronary Risk Prediction Chart. (March 2007) In *British National Formulary*. British Medical Association and Royal Pharmaceutical Society of Great Britain, London.

National Institute of Health and Clinical Excellence (NICE). (September, 2002) *Inherited clinical guidelines: management of type 2 diabetes. Management of blood glucose.* NICE, London.

National Institute of Health and Clinical Excellence (NICE). (October, 2002) *Inherited clinical guidelines: management of type 2 diabetes. Management of blood pressure and blood lipids.* NICE, London.

Prodigy guidance. (2007) *Diabetes glycaemic control.* www.cks.library.nhs.uk/diabetes_glycaemic_control/in_depth/management_issues Accessed on 27 February 2008.

Case 21 A 23-year-old woman with panic attacks

Miss Sewell, 23 years old, comes to see you. From the computer records you see that she was seen 2 weeks ago complaining of a lump in her throat. She was also seen by the 'out of hours' doctor last weekend complaining of difficulty in breathing. On both occasions the examination was recorded as normal and she was reassured.

You have not met her before and from her records you suspect the problem will be similar to before. When she comes in you note she is dressed with care and attention. She appears nervous with timid behaviour and poor initial eye contact. She is of mixed race.

She tells you that at night she feels that she cannot breathe, that it happens most nights and she feels there is something wrong.

What diagnoses spring to mind?
- Anxiety
- Panic attacks
- Depression
- Asthma
- Thyroid problems

What more specific questions would you like to ask?
- What specifically happens during the night?
- How long has it been going on?
- Any problems during the day?
- Any precipitation factors?
- How long do these feelings last?
- How does she control these feelings?
- Any associated symptoms?
- What specifically is she worried about?

Miss Sewell tells you that it has been going on for nearly a month and the 'attacks' are becoming more frequent. She holds her neck and says that she is unable to breathe, cannot get her breath and feels as though something is there. She says she has problems during the day but more commonly they occur at night. They generally happen when she is alone and when she is not occupied. The episodes last for 5–10 min, they end of their own accord and she is unable to control them. She reports that she can have palpitations, nausea and blurred vision. She is worried there is something wrong, causing her to have difficulty breathing and she worries what to do when this happens.

Is there any other relevant information that you would like to know?
- Medications, including over-the-counter medications
- Caffeine, alcohol, smoking and recreational drugs
- Social history, partner, job, family
- Any stressors?
- Past medical history

She takes the occasional paracetamol for period pains, drinks socially on the weekends, smokes 15 per day and denies taking recreational drugs. She lives alone in a flat, is of mixed race, is not in contact with her family and has friends from work. She works in a call centre for a bank. She denies any particular stressors but you feel she is of a generally anxious disposition. There is no specific past medical history.

What would you like to do next?
- Examination of cardiovascular system and thyroid
- Examination of mental state (Box 46)

On examination, she appears well and is not short of breath at rest, there are no signs of anaemia. She does appear nervous with a cautious nature and minimal responses to open questions. Her pulse rate is 80 beats/min and regular, BP 112/72 mmHg, heart sounds normal, chest clear, normal throat examination, no neck lumps palpable and no thyroid masses.

Mental state examination reveals her to be generally fidgety and she comes across nervously. She is meticulously dressed and you note much attention to detail and

PART 2: CASES

Box 46 Mental state examination

Performing this examination combines observation and asking questions to build a picture of the patient's current mental state. It requires you to step back and describe what is happening.

The format of the examination is:
- *Appearance and behaviour:* clothing, eye contact, rapport
- *Speech:* rate, form, content
- *Mood:* subjective – patient's description of their mood; objective – your view
- *Beliefs:* about their health
- *Hallucinations:* any unusual perceptions
- *Orientation:* time, place and person
- *Memory:* cognitive tests (e.g. date of birth, Prime Minister, monarch, count from 20–1)
- *Concentration:* on books, TV and reading, work
- *Insight:* awareness regarding their illness

---

a large shoulder bag with many papers and notes. She rates her mood as usually good but does get anxious at times, when alone and when her mind is not occupied. Her sleep is broken most nights but she can sleep through. She has good eye contact, is in a raised state of arousal and appears predominantly anxious. There is no suggestion of hallucinations or delusions. Her concentration is variable and at work it is good. Sometimes at home she reveals that she cannot concentrate well on reading. Her insight is limited by her preoccupation with the problem being a physical illness.

What is the differential diagnosis and reasoning?

1 *Anxiety, panic attacks or somatization:* this is the most likely explanation because of the episodic nature of panic attacks, the typical symptoms and normal examination. Also you have noticed that Miss Sewell seems to have an anxious disposition

2 *Asthma:* Miss Sewell's story is not a typical history of asthma. Examination is normal and there are no obvious precipitants such as allergens or exercise

3 *Thyroid disease:* this is not very likely as there is no tremor, hair loss, weight loss, diarrhoea, tachycardia or a palpable thyroid mass or swelling

What to do next?

You offer blood tests to rule out anaemia and her thyroid disease. A full blood count (FBC) and thyroid function

test (TFT) are requested. You direct her to the practice nurse for these tests.

You need to discuss with Miss Sewell the concerns she has for her health and how deep rooted the beliefs are that there is a physical reason for her symptoms. She needs to be reassured before she will fully accept that her symptoms may have a psychological origin.

After this discussion she tells you she fears that the lump in her throat may stop her breathing. You note that she truly believes in the presence of a throat lump. You reassure her that she does not describe symptoms of dysphagia, nor are there signs of a neck lump, stridor or wheeze. She reluctantly accepts this so you broach the idea of a psychological cause for her problems.

How would you reinforce the diagnosis?

To help this discussion you offer a leaflet (www.patient.co.uk) on panic attacks which supports your discussion that her symptoms relate to anxiety and panic and also contains a self-help guide which offers strategies to employ when an attack occurs.

You offer follow-up in 2 weeks to review the progress and allow for further discussion about the diagnosis (Box 47).

Box 47 Somatization

A process by which physical symptoms without adequate organic explanation are experienced and result in consultation (Gelder *et al.* 2001, p. 251)

Two week review

On review at the surgery Miss Sewell tells you that she has had two further episodes where she has felt unable to breathe. She is still convinced that there is a blockage. She tells you that she has read the leaflet that you gave her and she can see that some of the symptoms are indeed similar to her own experience. She seems only a little more comfortable at this appointment but you recognize that she is truly telling you her concerns which must not be dismissed.

How should you respond?

You seize this opportunity to tell her that you recognize how debilitating and distressing her problems are and reiterate that panic disorder is a spiralling feeling of raised anxieties based on fear of organic disease. You suggest that if she did have a blockage she would not have intermittent symptoms that resolve spontaneously, as in her case.

The use of time is a valuable tool in general practice. Symptoms and signs manifest over time. As described here with anxiety and panic attacks, discussion, negotiation and sharing understanding takes place over a number of consultations. You then reassure her that now the problems have been recognized, agreed and discussed, that it is entirely treatable and there are options open to her.

The conservative measures and lifestyle options include reducing caffeine and alcohol, addressing any workplace issues, increasing amount of exercise and enjoying a balanced healthy diet.

The NICE 2004 Anxiety guidelines recommend the prompt delivery of treatment, whether it be:
• Cognitive–behavioural therapy (CBT) – computer-based CBT, usual CBT
• Drug treatment – usually a selective serotonin reuptake inhibitor with panic disorder licence is first line therapy

Adherence to treatment is improved if the patient has been actively involved in the decision making and the services are available in the community. The counselling regarding medications is an essential part of the treatment plan. Best outcomes are achieved if the discussion involves:
• Awareness of early side-effects; including nausea and increased anxiety
• Discontinuation effects, particularly if treatment is stopped abruptly
• Awareness of the time delay before noticing improvements
• Duration of treatment: treatment is continued for a few months after the last symptom has resolved. This has been shown to reduce the risk of relapse, which can be up to 30% (Gelder *et al.* 2001, p. 240)

Treatment plans should be complemented with self-help guides and include advice regarding patient groups.

Following your detailed discussion with Miss Sewell, she decides upon a course of CBT. Pragmatically, this can take some weeks–months for an appointment to be available so you also offer short-term regular review with yourself to continue to develop the trust, offer advice and support.

CASE REVIEW

• Careful history-taking, clear understanding of attacks, their precipitants and how the attack terminates helps direct the differential diagnosis
• Physical examination aids to confirm the absence of pathology and reassures patients that their concerns are being taken seriously
• Mental state examination is important and allows some degree of objective assessment of the illness over time
• Understanding the timing of help-seeking behaviour (e.g. the use of services out-of-hours) points to aetiology and strategies can be employed to alter this behaviour
• Exploring the patients' ideas and beliefs is key to them having to change the view of their illness, from a physical to a psychological perspective
• Engaging with treatment depends upon the patients accepting the diagnosis and being involved in deciding upon the course of treatment
• Continuity of care was essential in this case. Trust had to develop between Miss Sewell and the doctor to allow her to move forward

KEY POINTS

• Anxiety and panic attacks are common problems
• Initial presentation as a physical illness is common (somatization) and it is often difficult to address the health beliefs of patients
• Establishing a therapeutic relationship allows trust to develop
• Use time as a therapeutic tool

References

Gelder, M., Mayou, R. & Cowen, P. (2001) *Shorter Oxford Textbook of Psychiatry*, 4th edn. Oxford Univeristy Press, Oxford.

National Institute of Health and Clinical Excellence (NICE). (2004) *Anxiety guidelines*. NICE, London.

National Institute of Health and Clinical Excellence (NICE). (2004) *Depression guidelines*. NICE, London.

Case 22   A 24-year-old woman who feels abnormally tired

Anita is a 24-year-old trainee accountant. You have little prior knowledge of her apart from seeing her a few months previously for contraception after she had a termination of pregnancy. She joined the practice earlier in the year when she moved into the area to start a new placement with an accountancy firm in the City of London. At the start of the consultation she sits down and describes how she has been feeling abnormally tired for the last few weeks.

What diagnostic possibilities spring to mind?

• She could simply be overworking – accountancy training is hard
• She may be suffering from stress that is unrelated to work
• She may have an organic disorder such as hypothyroidism or anaemia
• She may be depressed

You decide you need to know more and you let her talk freely for a few minutes, listening closely and observing her body language.

She tells you that she has been finding it difficult to get to sleep because work problems have been going round and round in her mind and even when she eventually drops off she has bad dreams. At work her concentration is poor and she has been recently working 10 h every day to complete everything. She says she feels she is useless, as she is always the last one to leave the office. Yesterday her boss shouted at her and she burst into tears in front of everyone else.

Although her clothes are smart, her hair is untidy and she is constantly fiddling with it and speaks in a monotone.

You are forming the impression that Anita is suffering from depression. What further information would be helpful at this stage to assess the severity of the condition?

• You need to ask about social support – does she live alone? How does she get on with her family?
• Get an idea about whether she has been enjoying any activities or interests outside work
• Whether she has suffered from depression in the past
• Whether anyone in the family suffers from depression
• Ask about appetite and weight
• Has she been feeling so bad that she has thought of harming herself?
See Boxes 48 and 49.

> **Box 48 Depression scoring systems**
>
> There are three commonly used depression scoring systems: the Beck Depression Inventory, the Hospital Anxiety and Depression scale and the PHQ-9. The PHQ-9 is commonly used in general practice. It uses nine items from the Diagnostic and Statistical Manual of Mental Disorders (DSM-IV) to score symptoms of major depression (Box 49).
>
> Depression questionnaires should not be used in isolation but as a useful adjunct to clinical assessment. It is not always appropriate to use them during the first consultation. The questionnaire can also be used repeatedly to monitor the patient's progress.

She tells you that she broke up with her boyfriend after the termination – that it was her decision and that he still keeps

> **Box 49 Diagnostic and Statistical Manual of Mental Disorders (DSM-IV) diagnostic criteria for a major depressive episode**
>
> For major depressive disorders, at least five of the following symptoms must be present most of the day, nearly every day for at least 2 weeks. At least one of the first two symptoms (in **bold**) must be present (NICE Guidelines on depression):
>
> 1 **Depressed mood**
> 2 **Markedly diminished interest in usual activities**
> 3 Significant increase/loss in appetite/weight
> 4 Insomnia/hypersomnia
> 5 Psychomotor agitation/retardation
> 6 Fatigue or loss of energy
> 7 Feelings of worthlessness or guilt
> 8 Difficulty with thinking, concentrating or making decisions
> 9 Recurrent thoughts of death or suicide

ringing her up. Her parents and two younger brothers live up North and she rings home once a week but does not like to worry them – her mother is on long-term antidepressants and her father has just had a bypass. They do not know she had a termination.

She is sharing a flat with two girlfriends who are aware that she is not quite herself and keep on trying to persuade her to go out but she has not felt like it because everything seems pointless. Normally a keen badminton player, she has not played for at least 3 weeks.

She had to resit her A-levels because she failed first time round and was rather low at that time. She saw a college counsellor who was very helpful when she was doing her degree in economics and geography.

She seemed to be both upset and relieved to disclose that she had in fact been thinking she would be better off dead, but she would not actually harm herself because it would hurt her parents too much.

What is your diagnosis and the reasons behind this? What do you say to Anita and what options are there for management?

You think she is probably suffering from reactive depression to overwork, moving house and a sense of loss after the break-up of her relationship and the termination.

She does not have the support of family close by. She has a family history of depression and may have had two or more episodes of depression previously. You ask her what she thinks would be helpful at this stage.

She says she would like to have herself 'checked out' in case there is something physically wrong with her. You agree to blood tests to check thyroid function and a full blood count. You say that you think that she is suffering from stress and depression and suggest she has some time off work. You reassure Anita that you expect her to get better and that you are sure you will be able to help her.

You ask her if she would like to try a course of antidepressants and whether she thinks she would like to have some therapy. You briefly describe what is involved in cognitive–behavioural therapy (CBT; Box 50) and give her a Mind leaflet. You refer her to the Mind website for further information about depression.

Anita is very determined to avoid antidepressants. She says she 'does not want to become addicted to them like my Mum is'. She is very worried about taking time off work but you persuade her to accept a certificate for 2 weeks and arrange to review her then. She is hoping that she will be able to catch up on sleep if she has some time off which will help her return to normal. From your clinical assessment you feel that she would benefit from antidepressants, but in your experience there is no point in insisting on this as you know that Anita will not take them if you give her a prescription. You make sure that she knows how to contact you in the meantime if she feels worse (Box 51). You ask her to complete a depression assessment questionnaire PHQ-9 in reception before she leaves.

> **Box 50 Cognitive–behavioural therapy (CBT)**
>
> - Trains the patient to learn to recognize and change negative thought patterns
> - Involves 'homework' for the patient in the form of exercises/diaries
> - Time-limited – usually 12–16 sessions
> - Based on current difficulties rather than analysis of past life
> - Encourages development of coping skills

> **Box 51 Learning points on initial management**
>
> - Rapport and reassurance that the patient will get better are important
> - Enable the patient to exercise her preferences for treatment
> - Watchful waiting
> - Close follow-up

Anita scored 17/27 on the questionnaire, confirming the diagnosis of moderately severe depression. You find Anita's old notes and see that she was bullied at school and was seen by a clinical psychologist just before she took her A-levels for the first time.

You are pleased to see Anita again 2 weeks later. You inform her that her blood tests are normal. However, her mood has worsened if anything, and she tells you that she is finding it difficult to be with other people and has hardly left the house. She is also finding it difficult to get out of bed in the morning and has been crying a lot of the time 'for no reason'. She has not arranged any therapy. She agrees to try a course of antidepressants saying, 'I'll try anything that might help me feel better'.

What issues do you need to consider when prescribing antidepressants?
See Box 52.

Box 52 When prescribing antidepressants

- Explain that they take 2–3 weeks to start working
- Reassure that they are not addictive
- Warn about common side-effects
- Choose antidepressant appropriately
- Prescribe in small amounts if the patient is suicidal to avoid overdosage
- Warn about discontinuation syndrome if the drug is stopped suddenly (symptoms of this include nausea, vomiting, chills, dizziness, agitation, impaired consciousness, fatigue)
- Arrange regular frequent review in the initial stages until the patient is in remission
- Explain length of course after remission

You arrange to see Anita 2 weeks later.

She has been taking 20 mg/day citalopram, and says she thinks she is feeling just slightly better, although she still is not sleeping and has started to worry about going back to work. She went up to Yorkshire to stay with her parents at the weekend and had a good talk with her mother which also helped.

You assure her that she will feel normal again but that it will take time and that she should have at least another month off work. You encourage her to arrange CBT with a local counsellor. Luckily she can afford to do this because the NHS clinical psychologist at the practice has a waiting time of 4 months.

You arrange to see her again in 3 weeks time and suggest some recommended self-help books on depression.

Three weeks later Anita is feeling much better. She is sleeping well and wants to return to work. She has been going out and playing badminton. She has more of a sparkle. She has started to see a counsellor who is helping her with negative thought patterns. She has also been working through the self-help book you recommended which she has found very useful.

You congratulate her and ask to see her in a month after her return to work.

The patient and her work
- Discuss when and how the patient should return to work. A gradual return is often best
- You may need to write a report for her employer
- The patient will need to give written consent and has the right to see the report.

Anita does not attend her next appointment with you. You write to her and ask her to come to see you again. When she does, she admits she ran out of her antidepressants 3 weeks previously and decided to stop them as she was feeling so well. You quickly discover that she has relapsed (Box 53).

Box 53 The importance of careful monitoring and follow-up

- Many patients stop their antidepressants when they feel better
- It can take several weeks for the antidepressants to come out of the system and for the patient to relapse
- Patients who do not attend need active follow-up

After this setback Anita decides to remain on the antidepressants and also completes 12 sessions of CBT. You continue to review her every 6 weeks and find it very rewarding that she continues to be well. Six months later she is enjoying work and has fallen in love. She comes to see you to discuss coming off the antidepressants (Box 54).

Box 54 What do you need to consider in the consultation regarding coming off the antidepressants?

- Discuss suitable timing to come off antidepressants. Some patients may wish to continue for longer than 6 months
- Devise a timetable for gradual tapering of the dose to avoid the discontinuation syndrome
- Depression scores can be useful to check for relapse
- Review the patient after they have stopped the antidepressants

This patient has an increased risk of further episodes, particularly during or after pregnancy because of her family history and her own history of previous depressive episodes. She will probably benefit from an annual review of her mood.

CASE REVIEW

Anita presented with abnormal tiredness which is a common symptom of depression. This was precipitated by a series of life events: she had recently moved house, started a new job, had a termination of pregnancy and broken up with her boyfriend. She is a vulnerable individual with both a past history of depression and a family history of the condition. Initially she is very unwilling to recognize that she needs treatment for clinical depression. You provide reassurance and support, certify her unfit for work, and follow her up closely. Her depression deepens and she recognizes that she needs help. As the depression begins to lift in response to antidepressant therapy, she is able to benefit from CBT. When she is feeling better she comes off the antidepressants and relapses. You make sure you follow her up and she recovers well from this episode. She will remain vulnerable to depression in the future.

KEY POINTS

- Patients with depression benefit from good support and continuity of care
- Depression questionnaires are a useful tool in diagnosis and monitoring
- Frequent follow-up is necessary to ensure compliance and to check treatment is successful
- Many patients are very unwilling to take antidepressants. Careful explanations are necessary when antidepressants are prescribed
- A combination of CBT and antidepressants have a good outcome for moderate depression
- Recurrent depression is common and it is therefore recommended that patients with a history of depression should be reviewed annually

References

National Institute for Health and Clinical Excellence (NICE). (2007) *Depression: Management of depression in primary and secondary care.* Clinical guideline No. 23 (amended). http://www.nice.org.uk/nicemedia/pdf/CG23NICEguidelineamended.pdf Accessed on 26 February 2008.

MIND (National Association for Mental Health). www.mind.org.uk.

A 54-year-old woman with urinary frequency and hot sweats

Mrs Kavorski is a 54-year-old woman who comes to the surgery rarely. She tells you that she keeps having to go to the toilet frequently in the day and once or twice at night. She also has hot sweats that wake her up and she feels tired most of the time. She thinks this is affecting her work as a supermarket manager as she has noticed her concentration is poor and she is irritable and 'not herself' at all.

What further questions would you ask her?

- How long have her symptoms been going on?
- When was her last period?
- Does she have any other urinary symptoms such as dysuria (burning) which might suggest an infection, or leakage of urine on coughing, laughing or sneezing (stress incontinence)?
- Has she ever had to get to the toilet quickly or not had time to get to there on occasion (urge incontinence)?
- Has she noticed any other problems such as feeling depressed or a low libido?
- Has she had children and any difficult deliveries with urinary problems subsequently?
- How did she think you might help?

Mrs Kavorski says she is not sure when her symptoms started but she thinks it was a few months ago. Her periods have been erratic for a couple of years and she has not had any periods in the last 10 months. She does not have pain on passing urine but seems to have to go more often than in the past. She does not have any problems with leaking urine when coughing, sneezing or getting to the toilet in time. She denies feeling depressed, just irritable and tired.

Her libido is definitely less than in the past but her husband has had diabetes for several years with erectile dysfunction so sex has been difficult and infrequent for a long time. She does have vaginal dryness on the few occasions they have tried intercourse. She has had three children – all normal deliveries and no problems afterwards.

She is not sure how you can help. She had wondered about hormone replacement therapy (HRT) but knows there are side-effects and risks attached to taking it.

What examination would you like to carry out and why?

- Blood pressure and weight (if raised this will influence your decision about treatment)
- Breast examination and cervical smear if these have not been carried out recently (currently cervical smears are performed every 5 years in women over 50 years up to age 65 years)
- Vulval and pelvic examination to assess state of the tissues and muscle tone
- Urinalysis to exclude diabetes and infection

Mrs Kavorski's blood pressure is 126/80 mmHg. Her weight is 66.3 kg and height 1.65 m which makes her body mass index 24.4 (which is in the normal range of 20–25). She had a normal cervical smear test 18 months ago and mammography 8 months ago which was negative.

Before you carry out any further examination you should offer to fetch a chaperone. Mrs Kavorski is happy to have one of the practice nurses there as well.

The breast examination is normal and there is no lymphadenopathy. When you examine the vulva you notice that the tissues are thin and shiny, indicating a degree of vaginal atrophy. There is no leakage of urine when you ask Mrs Kavorski to cough. Pelvic examination is unremarkable with a small anteverted uterus and no adnexal tenderness or masses. Vaginal tone is lax.

The practice nurse informs you that urinanalysis is negative for blood, protein, nitrites, leucocytes and glucose.

What are you going to say to Mrs Kavorski about your findings?

You can reassure her that you have not found anything seriously wrong and that her urine looks clear with no sign of infection or diabetes. The most likely cause for her symptoms of hot flushes and urinary frequency are her reduced levels of oestrogen due to the menopause. You explain to her that the tissues of the urinary tract are also oestrogen-dependent so it is common to have urinary symptoms at this time of life.

Mrs Kavorski asks if she can have a blood test to confirm that she is menopausal.

What blood tests would be taken to see if someone is menopausal and is it appropriate in this case?

You can measure follicle stimulating hormone (FSH) and luteinizing hormone (LH) levels which will be substantially raised in women who are menopausal. However, the blood test will not change your management and Mrs Kavorski has given a clear history of infrequent periods, urinary symptoms and hot flushes which suggest she is menopausal and further confirmation is not necessary.

You explain to Mrs Kavorski that her symptoms mean she is definitely going through the menopause and a blood test will not alter the options for treatment.

What treatments might you discuss with her?

• Topical oestrogens for her vaginal and urinary symptoms – this will not treat her hot sweats but will help with dryness and urinary frequency
• HRT – this will relieve both her hot sweats and urinary symptoms. It can be taken as tablets, transdermal patches or gel, nasal sprays or implants
• Tibolone tablets – a synthetic compound which combines oestrogenic and progestogenic activity with weak androgenic activity. It will relieve hot flushes and some urinary symptoms. (It is not suitable for women within 12 months of their last menstrual period because of irregular bleeding [*BNF* 2007]).

As Mrs Kavorski has not had a hysterectomy, if she decides to use HRT she will need a combined regimen of oestrogen and progestogen, rather than unopposed oestrogen which might lead to endometrial hyperplasia and an increased risk of cancer.

What else should you ask Mrs Kavorski before prescribing any hormonal therapy?

• Does she smoke?
• Is there any family history of breast cancer, bowel or ovarian cancer or premature heart disease?

• Has she ever had a clot in the leg or chest (deep vein thrombosis [DVT] or pulmonary embolism)?
• Has she ever had any problems with angina or symptoms that suggest peripheral vascular disease?
• Has she ever had liver disease?
• Has she had any unexplained vaginal bleeding?

You can see from her notes that she has not been treated for any malignancy in the past.

Mrs Kavorski has never smoked and there is no family or personal history of breast cancer, a deep vein thrombosis or pulmonary embolus. She has never had any problems with her liver. She has not had any cardiovascular problems but mentions that her twin sister (non-identical) has osteoarthritis.

You can reassure her that osteoarthritis is not a contraindication to HRT.

Mrs Kavorski says she has heard 'awful things' about HRT and is worried about developing breast cancer.

What are you going to say to her about the risks involved in taking HRT and specifically the risk of developing breast cancer?

It is important that you are well informed and take her concerns seriously as there has been much confusion about the risks of taking HRT following large studies in both the UK and the USA (Million Women Study Collaborators 2003; Women's Health Initiative 2002).

You say to Mrs Kavorski that currently studies have shown that there is only a *small* increase in risk of developing breast cancer if HRT is taken for a short time such as 1–3 years. The risk of breast cancer does increases with duration of use of HRT. Data from recent randomized controlled trials showed that this did not start to increase until 4 years after starting combined HRT (Prodigy Guidance on Menopause). There is some controversy about this because the Million Women Study suggested the risk starts to increase after 1–2 years, but experts have questioned the study because many of the women had been taking HRT for several years before entering the study.

You can tell Mrs Kavorski that there is probably only a small increased risk of breast cancer for women taking tibolone and it is less than for combined HRT. With all HRT preparations, the risk of breast cancer begins to decline when HRT is stopped and, by 5 years, it reaches the same level as in women who have never taken HRT

(CSM 2003a). There is also a small increase in the risk of stroke, clot, ovarian cancer and heart disease in women who take HRT compared to those who have never taken it, but Mrs Kavorski's medical history does not suggest she would be particularly susceptible to any of these complications.

Mrs Kavorski still looks very unsure about taking HRT and says she has heard of some 'natural' remedies for the menopause such as red clover and black cohosh and she wonders if these might be an alternative?

Many complementary therapies that are found in health food shops or sold on the Internet for the relief of menopausal symptoms contain phytoestrogens which are structurally similar to oestradiol, but there is little information available about their efficacy or safety. Currently, they cannot be recommended and some can be toxic to the liver (Ernst 2001; Huntley & Ernst 2003; ICSI 2003). Soya foods may help hot flushes and there are no known side-effects.

Mrs Kavorski has not asked about the benefits of HRT. Should you discuss these with her?

It would be a good idea to mention the fact that HRT will relieve her hot flushes, disturbed sleep, vaginal dryness and urinary symptoms. It also protects against thinning of the bones and colorectal cancer. Some women with osteoarthritis and joint pain find HRT helpful, perhaps because oestrogen has a role in the maintenance of collagen. As she is clearly not sure about whether she wants to try HRT, you decide to give her some written information to take away and suggest that she makes another appointment with you in a couple of weeks to discuss what she wants to do (Prodigy Guidance).

What other remedies might you suggest to Mrs Kavorski that do not involve medication?

- Regular exercise
- Lighter clothing
- Sleeping in a cooler room
- Reducing stress if possible

All of these measures may be helpful in managing hot flushes for many women plus the avoidance of possible triggers, including spicy foods, caffeine, smoking and alcohol. Unfortunately, they are unlikely to help with her urinary symptoms.

Follow-up

Mrs Kavorski comes back to see you in 2 weeks and says she would like to discuss topical oestrogen treatment because she has read that this is less risky than taking tablets or patches of HRT.

You can confirm this by reassuring her that the amount of oestrogen absorbed topically is minimal, so the risk of breast cancer is very low. When you check in the *British National Formulary*, you find you can prescribe either vaginal cream, tablets or pessaries or an Estring vaginal ring.

Mrs Kavorski does not like the idea of having a ring inserted so she opts for using the vaginal tablets. You instruct her that these should be used every night for 2–3 weeks and then reduced to twice weekly.

How long should she go on using topical treatment and should you warn her about symptoms such as vaginal bleeding that would warrant further investigation?

The Committee on Safety of Medicines (2003b) has advised that:

- Treatment should be interrupted at least annually to reassess the need for continued treatment
- If breakthrough bleeding or spotting appears at any time on therapy, this should be investigated possibly with endometrial biopsy to exclude endometrial malignancy

Does she need to take progestogens as well to protect against endometrial cancer?

Studies have found no significant association between the use of low-potency vaginal oestrogens and the relative risk of endometrial cancer (Weiderpass *et al.* 1999a). Expert consensus is that addition of a progestogen is not necessary for endometrial protection.

You prescribe 30 Vagifem tablets (oestradiol 25 μg in disposable applicators) and arrange to see Mrs Kavorski again in 6 weeks for review. You tell her that it can take several months and sometimes up to a year of treatment to alleviate symptoms. You are aware that topical oestrogen therapy will not relieve her hot flushes or poor sleep and that systemic HRT should still be an option in the future. You should arrange to check her blood pressure again in a year.

CASE REVIEW

New evidence is emerging all the time about the risks and benefits of HRT which can be confusing for both the public and the medical profession. In this case, Mrs Kavorski is worried about the risks of HRT and it is sensible to give her as much information as possible so that she can make an informed choice about the treatment (the Prodigy Guidance on Menopause website gives excellent information about all risks and benefits). For any individual considering HRT, a detailed history of symptoms, risk factors and preferences should be made and a discussion of lifestyle changes before any medication is given.

Atrophic vaginitis is common in postmenopausal women because of the decreasing levels of oestrogen. After the menopause, the decline in oestrogen and glycogen levels causes the pH of the vagina to rise and there is a proliferation of connective tissue, hyalinization of collagen and fragmentation of elastin (Semmens & Wagner 1982). The resulting thinning of the epithelium together with the fall in pH may result in infections, fissures and ulceration. These changes in the tissues also include the urinary tract because of the shared common embryologic origin. Vaginal and urethral epithelia are oestrogen-dependent and so both tend to thin and become more fragile when oestrogen levels decline.

As Mrs Kavorski's symptoms are mainly urinary frequency and nocturia and she is obviously anxious about the systemic effects of HRT, topical therapy is a good initial choice. Other women, particularly those who are sexually active, may prefer to choose oral or transdermal HRT to relieve their symptoms.

KEY POINTS

- About 80% of women experience menopausal symptoms, and 45% of them find the symptoms distressing (RCPE 2003).
- Although menopausal symptoms are usually self-limiting (2–5 years), some women experience symptoms for many years.
- Approximately 40% of women in the postmenopausal years will experience some of the symptoms of atrophic vaginitis; however, it is thought that only 20–25% of these will seek medical attention (Pandit & Ouslander 1997).
- The majority of women who chose to use HRT take it for 1–3 years and can be reassured that the increased risks of breast and ovarian cancer, stroke, DVT and heart disease are small compared to the benefits of HRT (e.g. relief of symptoms, prevention of osteoporosis)
- Many women do not need HRT, experience mild symptoms at the menopause and do not need treatment beyond reassurance and information including lifestyle advice
- Some women have distressing symptoms which interfere in a major way with their lives
- Before HRT is prescribed, the risks and benefits must be weighed up on an individual basis
- The route and preparation of HRT should be tailored to the individual
- The risk of breast cancer is increased by HRT but is still relatively low if HRT is taken for less than 4 years
- Other preparations besides HRT can be used to relieve some symptoms (tibolone, clonidine, selective serotonin reuptake inhibitors, vaginal lubricants such as K-Y Jelly)
- The role of complementary therapies and foods is unknown for the relief of menopausal symptoms; some preparations are hepatotoxic

References

British National Formulary. (2007) British Medical Association and Royal Pharmaceutical Society of Great Britain, London.

Committee on Safety of Medicines (CSM). (2003a) HRT: update on the risk of breast cancer and long-term safety. *Current Problems in Pharmacovigilance* **29**, 1–3.

Committee on Safety of Medicines (CSM). (2003b) Topical and vaginal oestrogens: endometrial safety. *Current Problems in Pharmacovigilance* **29**, 3.

Ernst, E. (2001) *Desktop Guide to Complementary and Alternative Medicine.* Mosby, London.

Huntley, A.L. & Ernst, E. (2003) A systematic review of herbal medicinal products for the treatment of menopausal symptoms. *Menopause* **10**, 465–476.

ICSI. (2003) *Health care guideline. Menopause and hormone therapy (HT): collaborative decision-making and management,* 5th edn. Healthcare Guideline. ICSI, Bloomington, MN.

Million Women Study Collaborators. (2003) Breast cancer and hormone-replacement therapy in the Million Women Study. *Lancet* **362**, 419–427.

Pandit, L. & Ouslander, J.G. (1997) Postmenopausal vaginal atrophy and atrophic vaginitis. *American Journal of the Medical Sciences* **314**, 228–231.

Prodigy guidance. http://cks.library.nhs.uk/patient_information_leaflet/menopause http://cks.library.nhs.uk/patient_information_leaflet/hormone_replacement_therapy

Prodigy guidance. *Menopause.* http://cks.library.nhs.uk/menopause/view_whole_guidance Accessed on 22 May 2007.

Royal College of Physicians of Edinburgh (RCPE). (2003) Consensus conference on hormone replacement therapy, October 2003. Final consensus statement. www.rcpe.ac.uk

Semmens, J.P. & Wagner, G. (1982) Estrogen deprivation and vaginal function in postmenopausal women. *JAMA* **248**, 445–448.

Weiderpass, E., Baron, J.A. & Adami, H.O. (1999) Low-potency oestrogen and risk of endometrial cancer: a case–control study. *Lancet* **353**, 1824–1828.

Women's Health Initiative. (2002) Risks and benefits of estrogen plus progestin in healthy postmenopausal women. Principal results from the Women's Health Initiative randomized controlled trial. *JAMA* **288**, 321–333.

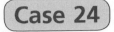

Case 24 A 19-year-old woman with vaginal discharge

Imogen Philips presents with a 2-week history of vaginal discharge. She is 19 and has no significant past medical history. She attends with Gemma, a friend from college. Imogen usually only attends the surgery to get her repeat prescription for the contraceptive pill.

What is the differential diagnosis for vaginal discharge?

See Box 55.

> **Box 55 Differential diagnosis for vaginal discharge**
>
> - A gynaecological infection:
>   - non-sexually transmitted: bacterial vaginosis, vulvovaginal thrush (*Candida*)
>   - sexually transmitted: *Chlamydia*, gonorrhoea, genital warts, genital herpes, syphilis, pelvic inflammatory disease, *Trichomonas*
> - Foreign bodies (e.g. retained tampons)
> - Malignancy

What questions do you need to ask?

- What is the duration and type of discharge?
- Is it offensive? If so, it would suggest bacterial vaginosis, *Trichomonas vaginalis* or foreign body
- Is there any vulval itching or vulval pain associated? If so, this would suggest *Candida*, *Trichomonas vaginalis*, bacterial vaginosis or herpes simplex
- Is the patient generally unwell?

She says that she has had several weeks of a thick discharge that has not been offensive and some mild lower abdominal pain but no vulval symptoms. She has not been generally unwell.

What other important information do you need to find out?

As some of the important differential diagnoses are sexually transmitted infections you need to ask if the patient is sexually active.

| *She looks a little embarrassed but says that she is.*

What other questions do you need to ask about her sexual history?

See Box 56.

> **Box 56 Components of a sexual history**
>
> Carter *et al.* (1998):
> - Social context and relationships
> - Contraception
> - Pregnancy and associated problems
> - Genital tract pathology (e.g. past sexually transmitted infections)
> - Sexual health promotion

Communication skills are paramount here. The questions should not be seen as a list that you need to go through. Handle them with care and tact. Be aware of your own attitudes and also of any cultural or language issues that may of importance (Carter *et al.* 1998). Possible questions to ask are covered by the Royal College of General Practitioners Handbook (Carter *et al.* 1998) but may include 'Are you in a sexual relationship?'; 'How long have you been together?'; 'Do you have any other partners?'

Imogen says that she has been with her boyfriend Mark for a couple of years. She has had no other sexual partners during that time but is worried because Gemma has heard that he has been 'sleeping around'. She thinks that she might have an infection that is causing her discharge and that is why she has come today.

PART 2: CASES

Why is Gemma with her?

She could be there to offer Imogen moral support or she could have been there as her partner. Another possibility is that Gemma insisted on it to make sure that her friend attended the doctor. Whatever the reason, you need to check whether the patient wants a third party to be present for the history or examination.

Apparently Gemma is here to support her and Imogen says that she wants her to stay throughout the consultation. Imogen is obviously upset with the information that she has just disclosed and so you allow some time for Gemma to comfort her.

What are your treatment options for a suspected sexually transmitted infection?

• Examination including taking the appropriate swabs and treatment depending on the results
• Referral to the local genitourinary medicine clinic
• Treatment blindly with antibiotics

   The most appropriate of these is referral to the clinic as they are specialists in providing appropriate support and contact tracing.

What form of history and examination should be carried out if she refuses to attend the clinic?

• Take a sexual history as outlined above
• Perform an abdominal and bimanual examination
• Take endocervical swabs for gonorrhoea and *Chlamydia*
• Take vaginal swabs for *Trichomonas*, *Gardnerella* and *Candida*

   Remember, if you do not test for it, you will not find it, and that multiple infections are common.

She refuses to go to the clinic and wants you to treat her. On examination, she has a mucopurulent discharge coming from an inflamed cervix. When you take the endocervical swabs there is a little contact bleeding. You also take a vaginal swab. There is no tenderness on bimanual or abdominal examination and there are no other positive findings.

What is the most likely diagnosis?

Chlamydia (Box 57).

What is the appropriate treatment?

Azithromycin 1 g as a single dose. This is in an effort to ensure good compliance although azithromycin is more expensive than the alternatives of doxycycline (7-day course) or erythromycin (14-day course; *BNF* 2006). You ask her to attend to discuss the swabs' results in a week's time.

The swabs confirm that she has Chlamydia infection and nil else.

What should you do next?

You should advise her of the diagnosis and check that her symptoms have resolved. You advise that she should attend the genitourinary medicine clinic to confirm that she has no other coexisting infections and also so that her partner and his contacts are traced for treatment if required.

Imogen was reluctant last time to go to the clinic what could you say to persuade her to attend now?

You could reinforce that the clinic is confidential, has specialist doctors and nurses who can diagnose and treat infections with appropriate contact tracing for partners. You could also explain that she could become reinfected if Mark is not treated and then she would be at further risk of complications.

What are the complications of *Chlamydia* that you should tell her?

See Box 58.

Box 57 Symptoms of *Chlamydia*

Coyne & Barton (2006):
• Purulent vaginal discharge
• Lower abdominal pain
• Postcoital bleeding
• Intermenstrual bleeding
• In men, dysuria and urethral discharge can occur

Box 58 Complications of *Chlamydia* infection

Drife & Magowan (2004); Jones & Boag (2007):
• Bartholin's gland abscesses
• Endometritis
• Salpingitis leading to tubal blockage, chronic pain and infertility
• Epididymo-orchitis in men
• It can also be passed on to the neonate

The consultation is drawing to a close when she blurts out that she is very nervous of telling Mark about the infection as the relationship is not going well anyway and she thinks that by divulging about the infection this will be the final straw.

You explain that the clinic could contact Mark for her if she feels unable to discuss it but by having an open chat about it she can ensure that he does seek treatment and therefore does not put her at risk of reinfection.

Is there any other information that she should have?

She should be advised to abstain from sexual intercourse until she and Mark have both been assessed and treated. This is also a good time to discuss her contraception.

She is currently using the combined pill only and has had no problems with this.

Is this the most appropriate form of contraception for her?

The combined pill is good for preventing pregnancy, when taken correctly, but will not protect against sexually transmitted infections. Best practice would be to advise her that she should use condoms as the best protection along with her combined pill.

Outcome. You provide her with written information about Chlamydia and write a letter of explanation for her to take to her appointment at the genitourinary medicine clinic. Imogen has a frank discussion with Mark telling him that she has Chlamydia and confronts him about his affair. He admits that he has had a relationship with someone else for the last few months and they decide to separate. He agrees to attend the clinic to be tested and treated.

Imogen has no side-effects from treatment and recovers without any problems. She then comes to you to ask about her future fertility as she understands that this could have been affected by the infection. You advise her that tubal blockage is unlikely as she had no signs or symptoms of ascending infection but that in the future if she is having problems conceiving this could be investigated.

CASE REVIEW

Presentation with sexually transmitted infection can be complex. Patients can present with many different symptoms that may not initially indicate an infection. For instance cystitis symptoms can be caused by urethritis from *Chlamydia*, gonorrhoea or *Trichomonas*. Abnormal vaginal bleeding can be caused by cervicitis from *Chlamydia* or gonorrhoea. Vaginal discharge can be caused by infection that is sexually or non-sexually transmitted but it can also be caused by other pathologies as indicated above.

Taking a sexual history can be embarrassing initially. The Royal College of General Practitioners handbook has many helpful suggestions of questions that can be used. Patients are unlikely to be embarrassed if you are not.

Chlamydia is the most common sexually transmitted infection diagnosed in the UK, there were 110,000 cases in 2005 (HPA 2006) and the number of cases is steadily rising. A national chlamydial screening programme has been introduced to offer opportunistic testing to all men and women under 25 years old. Its phased implementation began in 2001.

Best practice is to encourage patients with suspected sexually transmitted infection to attend the genitourinary medicine clinic. Besides being experts in treatment and diagnosis they are confidential and are experts in contact tracing (see below). They are also an excellent source of information and have specialist nurses who can take time to discuss things with her.

Partner notification (or contact tracing) is a process where the sexual partners of patients diagnosed with a sexually transmitted infection are informed of their exposure and the need to attend for a sexual health check. The aim is to prevent reinfection of the index case and to reduce the spread of infection, as they may be asymptomatic even though they are infected. Leaving the index case to inform the patient himself or herself may result in fewer patients presenting for a check-up than if the clinic or health care professional contacts them. If it is carried out this way, the index case's identity can be kept confidential (Mathews *et al.* 2001). Failure to treat the partners is probably the most common cause of treatment failure in *Chlamydia* infection (Gilson & Mindel 2001).

No one test is perfect and the majority of cases are asymptomatic; therefore this facilitates onward transmission. The advent of non-invasive tests is making asymptomatic screening more acceptable (e.g. urine tests or self-taken vulvovaginal swabs compared with endocervical swabs in women and urethral swabs in men; Coyne & Barton 2006).

KEY POINTS

- Differential diagnosis of vaginal discharge includes: gynaecological infection – non-sexually transmitted and sexually transmitted; foreign bodies (e.g. retained tampons); malignancy
- *Chlamydia* is the most common sexually transmitted infection in the UK
- Most cases of *Chlamydia* are asymptomatic but symptoms in women include: purulent vaginal discharge, lower abdominal pain, postcoital bleeding and intermenstrual bleeding
- Treatment should include patient education, antibiotics and contact tracing along with general contraceptive advice

References

British National Formulary, 52nd edn. (2006) Royal Pharmaceutical Society of Great Britain. RPS Publishing and BMJ Publishing Group, London.

Carter, Y., Moss, C. & Weyman, A. (eds.) (1998) *RCGP Handbook of Sexual Health in Primary Care.* Royal College of General Practitioners, London.

Coyne, K. & Barton, S. (2006) STIs. *Update* **72**, 11–20.

Drife, J. & Magowan, B. (ed.) (2004) *Clinical Obstetrics and Gynaecology.* Elsevier, London.

Gilson, R.J.C. & Mindel, A. (2001) Recent advances: sexually transmitted infections. *BMJ* **322**, 1160–1164.

Health Protection Agency (HPA). (2006) *A complex picture, HIV and other sexually transmitted infection in the United Kingdom.* Health Protection Agency. http://www.hpa.org.uk/publications/2006/hiv_sti_2006/contents.htm Accessed on 21 March 2007.

Jones, R. & Boag, F. (2007) Screening for chlamydia trachomatis. *BMJ* **334**, 703–704.

Mathews, C., Coetzee, N., Zwarenstein, M., *et al.* (2001) Strategies for partner notification for sexually transmitted diseases. *Cochrane Database of Systemic Reviews* Issue 4. Art. No.: CD002843.DOI:10.1002/14651858. CD002843.

PART 2: CASES

Case 25   A 34-year-old woman with 'funny periods'

Julia attends the surgery with 'funny periods'. She is fed up with not being able to predict when her period is due and has had prolonged spotting this month which was the 'final straw'. She looks a bit tired but not distressed.

She has not attended the surgery for many things in the past, other than moderately severe acne and an ankle sprain 2 years ago that necessitated some time off work. She is a secretary at the local brewery.

What might be the reasons why someone would attend with a menstrual bleeding problem?

After O'Flynn (2006):

• Some women think that their cycle is non-predictably irregular if their cycle only varies by 2–3 days and find this unacceptable
• The heaviness of acceptable menstrual bleeding varies widely
• In some religions prayer is not allowed when they are bleeding, making prolonged bleeding very problematic
• Fertility is often the most important factor in Julia's age group
• Many women worry that an irregular bleeding pattern indicates the menopause
• Julia may also be worrying about a specific pathology

What questions do you need to ask when completing a menstrual history?

See Box 59.

These questions should be handled sensitively, particularly as it is a topic that is treated as 'taboo' by some people.

Julia has had irregular bleeding for a year. Her cycle tends to be long with approximately 35–42 days between periods although she has not kept an exact diary. She bleeds for up to 12 days each cycle although she spotted for longer than that this last month. She has flooding and clots with

---

> **Box 59 Components of a menstrual history**
>
> National Collaborating Centre for Women's and Children's Health (2007):
> • Ask about the nature of the bleeding
> • Ask about related symptoms
> • Ask about the impact on the quality of life
> • Ask about the patient's ideas concerns and expectations
> • Date of last smear and previous results

associated pain at the beginning of each period but this tails off quickly. She has had intermenstrual bleeding on a couple of occasions and no postcoital bleeding.

She has not found her symptoms to be disabling and self-medicates with ibuprofen on occasion. Her main concern is that she has been trying to become pregnant for about a year now and is finding it difficult to predict when she is ovulating. Her husband also refuses to have intercourse if she is bleeding. There is no dyspareunia.

Her last smear was last October and it was normal. She has had no abnormalities in the past.

She wants to know what is the cause of her bleeding, if her bleeding is the reason why she has not become pregnant yet and if there is any way of controlling her bleeding without hormones.

What is the differential diagnosis for irregular menstrual bleeding?

See Box 60.

Do you have any other questions that you would like to ask her?

• When was her last period (helps to exclude current pregnancy)?
• What was her cycle like before these problems started?
• Has she any associated symptoms that might indicate a sexually transmitted infection?

PART 2: CASES

Box 60 Differential diagnosis for irregular menstrual bleeding

Elder (2002):
- Pregnancy related:
  - bleeding in pregnancy
  - retained products following miscarriage
  - ectopic pregnancy
- Anovulation:
  - anovulatory cycles related to menarche or menopause
  - pituitary or hypothalamus problems
  - polycystic ovary syndrome
  - thyroid dysfunction
- Malignancy:
  - endometrial
  - cervical
- Infection

Her last period started 2 weeks ago and she has not had unprotected intercourse since. Her menstrual irregularity started after she stopped taking the pill to try for a baby. She has had no pregnancies and has been on the pill since her early twenties. Prior to this her cycle had also been irregular.

She has had no vaginal discharge, dypareunia or history of sexually transmitted infection.

What examination would you like to perform?

You should carry out an abdominal and pelvic examination to complete your initial assessment.

Should swabs be taken to check for infection given the patient's history?

Sexually transmitted infections should be excluded in any patient who is sexually active who presents with menstrual problems as they are a possible cause and will not be detected unless tested for.

On examination, she is overweight, hirsute with excess hair on her face, lower abdomen and chest. She has a normal abdominal and pelvic examination. Swabs have been taken.

What is the most likely diagnosis?

You have ruled out pregnancy causes, malignancy is very unlikely and so anovulation is the most likely diagnosis although you will need to await the results of the swabs to confirm that she has no infection.

Explain why you should not be concerned about malignancy?

Age is a very important factor as carcinoma of the endometrium is very rare under the age of 35 years. Her smears are up to date and the cervix was of normal appearance on examination making cervical carcinoma highly unlikely. A change in status of symptoms is more likely to indicate pathology than those that have been present for a long time (Shapely *et al.* 2004).

What is the most likely cause of her anovulation?

She has features that are consistent with polycystic ovary syndrome (Box 61).

Box 61 Features suggestive of polycystic ovary syndrome

- Oligomenorrhoea
- Possible anovulatory infertility
- Hirsuitism and central obesity

What investigations would you perform to confirm polycystic ovary syndrome and what would be the expected findings?

See Box 62.

Box 62 Investigations for polycystic ovary syndrome

Drife and Magowan (2004); Thistlethwaite (2004):
- Ultrasound – bilaterally enlarged ovaries with multiple peripherally situated cysts. However, ultrasound can be misleading as cysts are not always present
- Testosterone and aldrostenedione may be elevated
- Luteinizing hormone is higher than follicle stimulating hormone
- Low sex hormone binding globulin

How could you proceed with the consultation?

- Explain what you think about her symptoms and examination findings
- Discuss the investigations that you would like to perform and why

- Address her main concern (her fertility) and advise her that she should start taking folic acid to reduce the chance of neural tube defect if she does become pregnant

You explain to Julia that the combined pill was probably providing her with a regular bleed and how without it she would probably have always had an irregular cycle. You confirm that this may cause problems with her trying to conceive and so you need to carry out some investigations.

You say that you would like to arrange for some blood tests and an ultrasound scan to aid your diagnosis. You decide not to tell Julia about polycystic ovary syndrome until it is confirmed and you arrange to see her a month later with the results.

One month later. Polycystic ovary syndrome is confirmed and the swabs for sexually transmitted infection are negative.

How would you proceed?

You need to explain to her the diagnosis and explain how polycystic ovary syndrome is the most common cause of infertility and that it is caused by the ovaries failing to produce eggs (anovulatory infertility; Drife & Magowan 2004). There may be some cycles where an egg is being released but as the couple have been trying for so long without success she needs referral to a specialist clinic to investigate her and her husband further so that they can be offered options for treatment as indicated (Box 63). You should also give her information to read (www.patient.co.uk) and offer support to the couple.

Box 63 Treatment for polycystic ovary syndrome

Drife & Magowan (2004):
- The cycle can be controlled with the combined oral contraceptive
- Hirsuitism controlled with combined oral contraceptive or cyproterone acetate
- The anovulatory cycles that it causes can be treated by oral anti-oestrogen therapy, clomiphene, with a cumulative pregnancy rate of 81% after 12 months treatment

---

Julia is understandably upset and asks if there is anything that she can do to improve her chances of conceiving while waiting for the referral.

You should calculate her body mass index, measure her waist circumference and sensitively explain to her that weight reduction should help to correct hormone imbalance and promote ovulation as well as to reduce insulin resistance that also occurs in polycystic ovary syndrome (Drife & Magowan 2004).

Which other health care professionals could be involved?

- The practice nurse could educate her about how to eat healthily and exercise safely
- A dietitian referral would also be useful, but usually there is a considerable wait for this service

Outcome. Julia and her husband are placed on the infertility clinic waiting list, which is several months long, and they are currently waiting for their outpatient appointment. To complete the referral several other investigations are carried out, according to protocol, including semen analysis on her husband.

You continue to see Julia frequently over the coming months as she is very anxious about her chances of conceiving and needs your support.

CASE REVIEW

In the UK, the cultural norm is not to talk about menstruation and therefore this can lead to difficulties when trying to assess women with menstrual disorders. Women can feel unable to share concerns with others and therefore this can limit their ability to cope with even minor menstrual problems (O'Flynn 2006).

Beliefs arise from a patient's personal experience and from social, cultural and educational influences. The normal menstrual loss is 3–8 days with an average cycle length of 28 days (NCC for Women's and Children's Health 2007).

Polycystic ovary syndrome is the most common endocrine disorder in women of reproductive age (Kunde & Khallaf 2006). Its aetiology is not entirely clear although the key features are insulin resistance, androgen excess and abnormal gonadotrophin dynamics. One of the results is an anovulatory state and this in turn usually leads to a polycystic ovary (Hunter & Sterrett 2000). This occurs as the follicles start to develop but do not mature and become fluid-filled cysts. There is a tendency for it to run in families although the genetic component has not been identified.

There is a spectrum of presentation from mild to severe and therefore many women with the condition will not even present to their GP. Treatment depends on the presenting symptoms and on the priorities of the patient. In this case fertility was the most important factor and so Julia and her husband were referred to a fertility clinic.

KEY POINTS

- Reasons for women attending with menstrual disorders are inability to cope with their symptoms, concern about underlying pathology, concern about fertility or worries about the menopause
- The differential diagnosis for irregular menstrual bleeding includes pregnancy related causes, anovulation, malignancy and infection
- Polycystic ovary syndrome:
  - can present with menstrual oligomenorrhoea or amenorrhoea, central obesity and hirsuitism and acne
  - an ultrasound scan is not always diagnostic and so diagnosis can be confirmed from the history, examination and analysis of sexual hormones
  - treatment depends on the presenting symptom and the priority of the patient

References

Drife, J. & Magowan, B. (ed) (2004) *Clinical Obstetrics and Gynaecology.* Elsevier, London.

Elder, M.G. (2002) *Obstetrics and Gynaecology: Clinical and Basic Science Aspects.* Imperial College Press, London.

Hunter, M.H. & Sterrett, J.J. (2000) Polycystic ovary syndrome: it's not just infertility. *American Family Physician* **62**, 1079–1090.

Kunde, D. & Khallaf, Y. (2006) Key developments in women's health. *Practitioner* **250**, 7–13.

National Collaborating Centre for Women's and Child's Health Commissioned by National Institute for Health and Clinical Excellence. (2007) *Heavy menstrual bleeding.* http://guidance.nice.org.uk/CG44 Accessed on 5 April 2007.

O'Flynn, N. (2006) Menstrual symptoms: the importance of social factors in women's experiences. *British Journal of General Practice* **56**, 950–957.

Shapely, M., Jordan, K. & Croft, P.R. (2004) An epidemiological survey of symptoms of menstrual loss in the community. *British Journal of General Practice* **54**, 359–363.

Thistlethwaite, J. (2004) Key developments in menstrual problems. *Update* 161–174.

Case 26 A 15-year-old girl with a problem

Lisa Johnson is a 15-year-old girl (the daughter of Mr Johnson with indigestion, Case 14), whom you have know since she was at primary school. She rarely comes to see you, but arrives one Monday afternoon in her school uniform looking upset. When you ask her what is wrong, she bursts into tears and says she is pregnant and 'my Dad'll kill me'.

How would you respond to this situation?

• Stay calm and offer her some tissues
• Find out if she has done a pregnancy test
• Ask her how you can help and what she wants to do about the pregnancy
• Reassure her that the consultation is confidential and you will not tell anyone without her express permission

Lisa manages to stop crying enough to tell you that she has done two pregnancy tests at the chemist and they are both positive. She also has very sore breasts and is putting on weight. She is devastated to be pregnant and wants an abortion. She is terrified that you will tell her parents.

What do you need to ask Lisa about the situation?

• When was her last period?
• Is she having regular periods?
• How long has she been sexually active?
• Was she using any contraception – if so, what sort?
• Does she have a regular boyfriend?
• Was she raped?
• Is she certain that she wants a termination? What are the alternatives?

Lisa thinks her last period was about 8 weeks ago. She has always had irregular periods. She has had sex only on one occasion when she went to a sleepover at a friend's house and had too much to drink. She knew the boy she slept with slightly, but has not seen him since. It was not rape. He does not know she is pregnant. She did not use any

contraception. She is adamant that she does not want to continue with the pregnancy.

What other things go through your mind given this information?

• Lisa may be at risk of acquiring a sexually transmitted disease
• She may be drinking too much alcohol on a regular basis and putting her health at risk
• She will need contraceptive advice in the future
• You are not sure where you stand legally about referring her for a termination as she is under 16 years. You are also unclear whether the father of the baby has any rights.

This is a complicated situation and some doctors are not willing to refer patients to have a termination because it is against their religious or ethical beliefs. If this is the case, GMC *Good Medical Practice* states that: 'If you feel your beliefs might affect the advice or treatment you provide, you must explain this to patients and tell them of their right to see another doctor.'

It would be sensible to get in touch with your medical defence organization for advice in this complex case. General Medical Council guidelines are that girls under the age of 16 years may be able to reach an informed decision depending on their capacity to comprehend everything involved in the procedure.

It is impractical to send Lisa away to come back later so you ask her to wait in your room while you go and ring your medical defence organization from another location.

The medical defence organization's advice is that you should try and persuade Lisa to talk to at least one of her parents about the pregnancy. However, if she refuses to do this, you must use your professional judgement to assess if Lisa is competent to understand the risks of having a termination, both to her physical and mental health. If you think she is competent, then you do not have to have

PART 2: CASES

Box 64 Epidemiology of abortion

In 2004, 185,400 terminations of pregnancies were performed on UK residents, a rise of 2.1% on 2003. This was equivalent to an age-standardized abortion rate of 17.8 per 1000 resident women aged 15–44 years. The highest age-standardized abortion rate in 2004 was 31.9 per 1000 women in the 18–19 and 20–24 age groups. The under-16 abortion rate in the same year was 3.7 compared with 3.9 in 2003. The under-18 rate was 17.8 compared with 18.2 in 2003. The NHS funded 82% of abortions in 2004; of these, just over half (51%) took place in the independent sector under NHS contract: 88% of abortions were carried out at under 13 weeks' gestation; 60% were at under 10 weeks. Medical abortions accounted for 19% of the total compared with 17% in 2003. Only 1% of UK abortions conducted in 2004 were on the grounds of a risk of severe mental or physical handicap in the child (Department of Health Abortion Statistics).

Legal requirements

The 1967 Abortion Act allows termination before 24 weeks if it:

- Reduces the risk to a woman's life
- Reduces the risk to her physical or mental health
- Reduces the risk to physical or mental health of her existing children, or
- The baby is at substantial risk of being seriously mentally or physically handicapped

Most terminations are performed under the second of these criteria.

---

parental consent before referring her to see a gynaecologist and you can sign the appropriate form (HSA1) requesting a termination. The gynaecologist also has to make his or her own assessment and agree to sign the form HSA1 before the operation can be carried out. As the law stands at the moment, the father of the baby does not have to be informed of Lisa's decision to have a termination.

As Lisa's GP, you will probably feel very uncomfortable with this situation. You should strongly encourage Lisa to confide in someone, preferably one of her parents, about what is going on. She is likely to need a lot of emotional support while going through this process and it would be much better if her mother or a good friend could help, as well as yourself. *Good Medical Practice* (GMC) states that: 'Medical professionals should try and facilitate a dialogue between child and parent. When this is not pos-

sible, the doctor needs to help find the young person an alternative means of support.'

Lisa is adamant that she is not able to tell either of her parents, but thinks she could confide in one good friend from school.

You strongly suggest that Lisa does talk to her friend and then ask if you can examine her.

What physical examination do you need to do today to sort out the situation?

- Blood pressure and weight
- Pelvic examination to confirm the size of the pregnancy
- Triple swabs for sexually transmitted diseases (two endocervical swabs, one for *Chlamydia* and one for gonorrhoea, and one high vaginal swab for other infections)

You must offer a chaperone for internal examinations so you ask the practice nurse to be present. This is particularly important if you are a male GP. If you are a female GP, you should still offer to have a chaperone but if Lisa declines this, document the fact in the notes.

When you examine Lisa, she has a thick white vaginal discharge and the uterus is the size of a large grapefruit (10–12 weeks' size), which makes an urgent gynaecology appointment necessary if she is to have a suction termination (Box 65). Her blood pressure is normal 100/66 mmHg and weight 59 kg.

What do you need to tell Lisa about having a termination?

You need to tell her briefly about the risks of the operation (failure rate – i.e. incomplete removal of the pregnancy, risk of bleeding, infection, perforation of the uterus; see Box 66) so that Lisa is fully informed. You can warn her that she is likely to feel upset after the termination, even though she is desperate to have it done, because she will probably feel guilty and worried about the consequences. These issues will also be discussed further at the gynaecology outpatient appointment. If you think Lisa understands all these issues, you may be willing to do the referral letter and sign the HSA1 form.

The emotional consequences of having a termination may be worse than the physical trauma and depression and guilt are very common.

Box 65 Abortion services

The availability of abortion services may vary geographically and be much more difficult to access in rural or remote areas of the UK. In some districts, the Primary Care Trusts are now commissioning charities such as the British Pregnancy Advice Services or the Marie Stopes Centres to carry out NHS terminations.

Different techniques of termination are practised depending on the gestation of the pregnancy:

- Medical abortion using a single oral dose of the antiprogesterone mifepristone followed by a single oral dose of a prostaglandin may be used up to 9 weeks' gestation. Medical abortion can also be used at later gestations, but requires multiple doses of prostaglandin to induce labour.
- Suction aspiration can by used below 7 weeks
- Suction termination with curettage under local or general anaesthetic is used between 7 and 15 weeks
- After 15 weeks, surgical dilation and evacuation by suction and specialized forceps

---

Box 66 RCOG estimates of risk

- *Failed abortion:* 2–3 in 1000 surgical abortion, 1–14 in medical abortion
- *Infection* (genital tract and pelvic inflammatory disease): approximately 10% and this can lead to infertility in the future
- *Haemorrhage:* 1 in 1000 overall but only 0.88 in 1000 if pregnancy is under 13 weeks
- *Uterine perforation:* 1–4 in 1000
- *Cervical trauma:* no more than 1 in 1000

All these figures depend on the skill and experience of the doctor performing the procedure.

Box 67 Information needed in the referral letter for a termination of pregnancy

- Name, date of birth and first day of last menstrual period or indication of how far the pregnancy has progressed (10–12 weeks in this case)
- Any relevant past medical history – Lisa is allergic to penicillin. No operations or serious illnesses
- Weight and blood pressure
- Social circumstances and reason why requesting a termination
- Your assessment of her competency to understand the procedure and take responsibility for her decision
- Contraceptive history (none)
- Your name, qualifications and contact details
- Form HSA1 filled in correctly

You should also mention that you have taken triple swabs and will fax through the results as soon as they are available.

She will need to take the referral letter and form and an early morning urine specimen with her (Box 67). At the appointment she will have an ultrasound scan to confirm the size of the pregnancy. If the pregnancy is less than 15 weeks, the gynaecologist will make arrangements to admit her as a day case as soon as possible. After the operation, she is likely to feel tired and upset. She will need someone to look after her and take her home later in the day (for more detail about termination procedures see Box 67).

You are conscious that your surgery is running 30 mins late and you cannot sort this all out now. You ask Lisa to call in to the surgery tomorrow to pick up the referral letter and form for the gynaecologist. You give her a patient information leaflet about having a termination and a urine specimen bottle.

What follow-up arrangements should you make?

You arrange to see Lisa again in a few days to give her the results of the triple swabs and see if she has managed to talk to her parents or a friend about the situation.

After your morning surgery has finished, you telephone the Fertility Control Unit at the hospital to arrange an urgent appointment for Lisa. Unfortunately, it is now lunchtime and there is only an answerphone service on which you leave a message asking them to call you back on your mobile telephone.

Lisa appears to take all this information on board and is still sure she wants to be referred for a termination.

If you are going ahead with the referral, what practical information does Lisa need to know?

You tell Lisa that you arrange an urgent outpatient appointment for her in the Fertility Control Unit (part of gynaecology) where she will be seen, examined, have a blood test and be counselled about having a termination. The decision about whether this will go ahead depends on the doctor who sees her at the hospital and whether they are also willing to sign the HSA1 form.

Later the same day

You are out on a home visit when the Fertility Control Unit ring you back. This puts you in a difficult position as you cannot talk to them without breaching confidentiality if you are with another patient. You tell them you will ring back in 10 mins when you have finished dealing with Mrs B., an elderly woman with dementia.

You call the clinic back from the privacy of your car and explain the urgency of the situation with Lisa. The gynaecology clerk is very helpful and says they will see her on Friday at 17.30.

Three days later

The triple swab results come back and are negative for *Chlamydia*, *Trichomonas* and gonorrhoea, but positive for *Candida* (thrush). Unfortunately, Lisa does not turn up for her 16.30 appointment with you. The receptionist confirms that she did come in to pick up the referral letter for the Fertility Control Unit the day before.

What treatment should you prescribe and how are you going to inform Lisa?

You could prescribe a clotrimazole pessary and clotrimazole cream 2% but if Lisa has never used these before she will need instruction. You could try telephoning her at home or sending her an urgent appointment through the post but some patients do not like receiving letters, particularly teenagers living at home. You regret not taking Lisa's mobile telephone number. Also, it is now Thursday and Lisa's hospital appointment is the next day. You decide to fax the swab results through to the Fertility Control Unit so they can prescribe and explain about the treatment when they see Lisa.

You need to see Lisa after the termination so you ask the receptionist to write to her asking her to make an appointment with you in about 2 weeks. This will not mention the reason for the consultation in case anyone else at home picks up the letter.

14 days later

You receive a discharge letter from the hospital informing you that Lisa has had the termination and the pregnancy was estimated to be about 13 weeks. Lisa arrives after school to see you later that day.

What questions do you need to ask Lisa at the appointment today?

- How is she feeling generally?
- Any pain or bleeding?

- Any vaginal discharge or itching?
- Does she need contraception?
- If she does want contraception, has she had unprotected sex since the termination?
- Whether she has confided in anyone since you last saw her?

Lisa tells you that she is feeling alright, although she looks anxious and as if she might burst into tears. She has not told her parents or any adult about the pregnancy. She stayed with a school friend after the termination who is the only other person who knows about the pregnancy. She did have some vaginal bleeding but this has now stopped. She has not had sex again. She was prescribed a month's supply of the oral contraceptive pill (Marvelon) at the hospital, which she has been taking regularly. She was given a tablet (fluconazole 150 mg) to get rid of the Candida infection preoperatively. She has not had any itching or vaginal discharge since.

What else do you need to ask her and what follow-up arrangements should you make?

- Is she depressed? To ascertain this you need to ask about specific symptoms such as her sleep pattern, appetite, view of the future and energy levels
- It would be sensible to offer to see her in a few weeks. She will need another prescription for the contraceptive pill with advice about what to do if she forgets to take it

Lisa is definitely upset and miserable. She is sleeping and eating all right and looking forward to 'everything being normal again'. She is still very anxious that her parents will find out what has happened. You do not think she is clinically depressed. She agrees to come back to see you in 3 weeks and takes the prescription for 3 months of the contraceptive pill with her, plus a supply of condoms.

Should you tackle the question about how much alcohol she is drinking and whether she is putting herself at risk generally?

This is an issue that needs exploring as Lisa may be drinking more than is sensible on a regular basis, which can lead to risky behaviour as well as being detrimental to her general health. At this appointment, you decide Lisa is not in a fit state to take in much information. You reassure her again that you will not tell anyone about what has happened. You talk in general terms about the fact that teenagers often drink too much alcohol and that the consequences can be devastating (e.g. risky sexual behaviour leading to pregnancy, sexually transmitted diseases, injury, liver problems). You ask her to think about these issues and give her a leaflet on safe drinking. You make her another appointment to see you again in 3 weeks.

CASE REVIEW

Unwanted pregnancy and the request for a termination raises many ethical and emotional issues for both the patient and the health professional. This is particularly the case when the patient is under 16 years. The General Medical Council Guidelines in Good Medical Practice are a useful reference guide for dealing with under-16-year-olds and your medical defence organization can also be very helpful. You must be very careful not to break confidentiality in a case like this and make sure you document each consultation meticulously.

If your own beliefs prevent you from treating a patient, you must explain this to them and ask them to consult another doctor, as you still have a duty of care to the patient.

In Lisa's case, there are three potential health risks that you must deal with:

1 Mental health risk of continuing or terminating the pregnancy
2 Risk of sexually transmitted disease following unprotected sex
3 Risk of drinking excessive alcohol

Follow-up is also crucial and counselling about contraception and sensible drinking to prevent any further unwanted pregnancies.

Chlamydia is detectable 7–10 days after exposure and Lisa is lucky not to have contracted this from her casual sexual encounter. According to the Health Protection Agency, genital chlamydial infection is currently the most common sexually transmitted infection (STI) diagnosed in genitourinary clinics in the UK and rates have risen steadily since the mid 1990s. A study by the Health Education Authority in 1998 showed 1 in 7 young people had unsafe sex after drinking alcohol and 1 in 10 had drunk so much they could not remember if they had had sex or not. As Lisa's GP, your role in advising about safe sex and moderate drinking is very important in preventing problems in the future.

This case also raises important points about how we should communicate with patients. Mobile telephones and email can make it easier to contact a person directly and, in the case of teenagers particularly, these can be good ways to get in touch and ensure privacy.

KEY POINTS

- An unwanted pregnancy and subsequent termination is a traumatic event and often followed by depression and guilt
- In all cases involving under-16-year-olds the GMC recommends that doctors encourage the patient to discuss the problem with their parents
- The medical defence organizations will provide advice on difficult ethical issues such as treatment and referral for the under-16-year-old patient
- Health education about 'safe sex' practices and using contraception effectively is a very important part of the GP's work when dealing with young people

- Maintaining confidentiality is crucial
- Documenting in the notes exactly what was discussed and agreed is particularly important in difficult ethical situations such as Lisa's
- You must maintain a non-judgemental stance and act in the patient's best interests at all times. This may include suggesting they see another doctor if your own religious or ethical views prevent you from referring a patient for a termination of pregnancy

References

Department of Health Abortion Statistics. www.patient.co.uk/showdoc/40000047 Accessed on 15 October 2006.

General Medical Council (GMC). (2006) *Good medical practice.* www.gmc-uk.org/guidance/good_medical_practice/index.asp Accessed 22 July 2007.

Health Education Authority/British Medical Research Board. (1998) *Sexual health matters: research survey.* HEA, London.

Health Protection Agency (HPA). http://www.hpa.org.uk/infections/topics_az/hiv_and_sti-chlamydia/default.htm Accessed on 22 July 2007.

Royal College of Obstetricians and Gynaecologists (RCOG). www.rcog.org.uk/resources/Public/pdi/abortion_summary.pdf Accessed on 13 October 2006.

Case 27 A 27-year-old pregnant woman with backache and anaemia

Fatima Khan is well known to you as she has seen you several times with recurrent depression. She is otherwise well and has not been on any medication for over a year. She is currently 26 weeks pregnant with her first child after trying to conceive for several years. She has come to see you today complaining of back pain.

Fatima and her husband Mo have been living with his parents since they got married 6 years ago. The family have been putting a lot of pressure on the couple to have a baby and so all were delighted when they found out about the pregnancy.

You saw her with some vaginal bleeding in early pregnancy but this settled quickly. She also had hyperemesis and fatigue during the first trimester and required 2 weeks off work to allow her to recover from her sickness. She works as a cleaner for a firm that cleans offices and works five evening shifts a week.

Her dating and anomaly scans, triple test, blood pressure and urinalysis have all been normal. She had borderline anaemia at her booking appointment but you are not aware of any more recent blood test results.

What are the two most common causes of back pain in pregnancy?

- Mechanical back pain
- Disc herniation

Disc herniation is rare but it should be suspected in patients with significant low back pain and those with neurological signs or symptoms (e.g. radiation down the sciatic nerve distribution). These patients should be referred urgently for investigation and treatment so that the chance of permanent neurological damage can be minimized (Garmel *et al*. 1997).

What questions would you like to ask her about the pain?

- How long has she had the pain?
- What is its character, site and radiation, in particular does it travel down her legs?
- Has she experienced pain like this before?

- Has she taken anything for the pain? Any precipitating or relieving factors?
- What does she think that the pain is caused by (often brings out irrational fears or gives you the diagnosis)?
- Has she any numbness or pins and needles in her legs or buttocks?
- Has she had any problems opening her bowels or urinating?

Fatima says that she has experienced an odd twinge in her lower back at work ever since she started work as a cleaner. Her pain normally settles when she rests, particularly when she has her days off at the weekends. She has now had pain constantly for several weeks. It is in the small of her back, aches and does not travel down her legs. She has had no pins and needles or numbness. She has no problems with urinating but she has been a little constipated throughout the pregnancy.

She has not been taking anything for the pain, as she did not think that she could take anything while pregnant. She thinks that work is making it worse and is worried that it might be affecting the baby.

What is the most likely diagnosis?

There is no indication of disc herniation and so this is most likely to be mechanical low back pain.

What factors make back pain common in pregnancy?

The mechanism for pain is not clear but an increase in joint laxity, symphysis pubis and sacroiliac joint changes have all been postulated (Brynhildsen *et al*. 1998) along with posture changes (National Collaborating Centre for Women's and Children's Health 2003).

Are there any other diagnoses that you would like to rule out? If so, what further questions would you ask?

Urinary tract infection

This is common in pregnancy and can present with back pain. Although she has said that she has had no problems urinating, ask her if she has had any pain on urinating or been needing to go more often than usual?

This is not likely, as she has not had any urinary symptoms and the urine sample that she had tested last week, during her routine appointment with the midwife, was recorded as normal.

Malingering

This presents with symptoms intentionally produced with the aim of securing tangible benefits (e.g. time off work; Fitzpatrick 2003). It is difficult to diagnose, particularly if you do not know the patient. You could find out more about what she might have to gain from the pain by asking questions about what happens at work or home when she has the pain.

This is unlikely in this case as Fatima does not even get sick pay when she needs to take time off work. At home her family does not give her any sympathy and she is still expected to do most of the household chores.

Although malingering is unlikely, it does not rule out a psychological component to her symptoms.

What is another possible psychological diagnosis?
Depression and anxiety

These often present with somatic symptoms (Mayou 2002).

This diagnosis is highly likely in this patient as she has seen you with depression in the past and she is under pressure both at work and at home.

How should you handle her back pain?

You should reassure her that the pain sounds like it is simple mechanical pain brought about by a strain in the muscles and ligaments of her lower back. You also need to explain that it is common in pregnancy as a result of the action of the hormones on the joints and also the change in posture. You can reassure her that it is OK to take some paracetamol for the pain during pregnancy.

Her specific concern with this was whether it was harming the baby so you need to reassure her that her pain should not have an adverse effect on the baby.

Fatima is relieved with the diagnosis and glad that you think that it should not harm the baby. She says that she would rather cope with the pain than take any medication.

You also decide to ask how things are at home at the moment and if she feels that her work is too much for her at present?

Things at home are pretty strained at the moment and so it is quite a relief to go out to work. She and her husband have been arguing about when they will be able to afford to buy a place of their own. There is not much room in his parent's house and she is worried that there will not be enough space for the baby to play when it starts crawling.

How could you introduce to her the fact that there may be a psychological component to her pain?

You say to her that you are sorry that there are so many stresses at home and that often people with these kinds of stresses can experience pain worse that those without.

She becomes upset as she thinks that you do not believe that she has any pain. You defend yourself by saying that you think the pain is very real and that you just think that the stresses are not helping her to cope with it.

She asks what else you can do other than offer more time off work as she cannot afford it.

What are effective treatments for back pain in pregnancy?

See Box 68.

> **Box 68 Effective treatments for back pain in pregnancy**
>
> NCC for Women's and Children's Health (2003):
> - Exercise in water
> - Massage therapy
> - Group or individual back care classes

You should also offer her reassurance, paracetamol and a follow-up appointment if things do not improve. Physiotherapy can also help through educating the patient about appropriate back care.

Having considered the options, you offer to refer her to the obstetric physiotherapist reassuring her that she sees a lot of pregnant women with back pain. You tell her that she will be assessed and given exercises to help relieve the pain.

She is dubious that exercise will help the pain but says that she might as well give it a go.

When you are writing in her handheld notes you notice that she had a follow-up haemoglobin (Hb) taken at her antenatal appointment last week. You look this up on the computer lablink system and find out that her Hb has fallen to 10.1 g/dL.

Why might she have a low Hb?

Many women have low iron stores and this can put them at increased risk of anaemia when they are pregnant. The normal physiological response in pregnancy can look similar and is due to a dilutional effect because of the increase in plasma volume.

Should you worry about Fatima's Hb?

The normal range is defined as Hb >11 g/dL at booking or >10.5 g/dL in the third trimester. Very low Hb is associated with poor outcome and so if a level outside the normal range is detected it should be investigated and iron supplements considered (NCC for Women's and Children's Health 2003).

I *Her iron level has also been measured and it is low.*

What should you do?

Explain that she is anaemic and that this could be contributing to her tiredness. Also, if it drops a lot further it could be harmful to her and the child.

Discuss her dietary intake of iron. Explain that it is found in meat, green vegetables (e.g. broccoli and spinach), cereals, strawberries and eggs. Vitamin C helps the body to absorb iron and is found in citrus fruits and cranberries, including their juices. Tea and coffee reduce the absorption of iron and so should be avoided. More information can be found from www.nhs.co.uk. You should also advise that although liver is full of iron it should be avoided in pregnancy because it is harmful to the baby.

Discuss the need for iron supplements and their possible side-effects (gastric irritation, nausea and altered bowel habit; *BNF* 2006). You could discuss the ways of reducing side-effects (Box 69). Constipation is common

---

> **Box 69 Ways of reducing side-effects from iron tablets**
>
> - Taking the tablets with meals, but food reduces the absorption of iron and so a longer course may be required
> - Taking a lower dose, but again a longer course may be required

---

in pregnancy and will be exacerbated by iron supplements, laxatives should be offered.

Outcome. Fatima starts to see the physiotherapist but finds this of little help and still complains of back pain throughout her pregnancy. She starts to take the iron tablets but these cause constipation and nausea so she stops them after a few weeks. At her follow-up appointment you negotiate with her that if her Hb has not dropped any further then she can leave out the supplements. It comes back as 10.4 g/dL and so you opt to recheck it monthly.

Fatima has a baby boy 3 weeks early. Mother and baby are kept in hospital for a week as she struggles to breastfeed him. Eventually, reluctantly, she decides to feed him on formula milk. She is followed up regularly by the midwife and health visitor as the team worry that she may develop postnatal depression. She manages well throughout the initial months caring for her new son.

Fatima comes to you 4 months after her son is born requesting sterilization. She says that does not want another child as the back pain was unbearable. You persuade her not to go for such a permanent form of contraception at this stage and offer her a coil with a promise that you will review the situation with her in 12 months. Her back pain continues to be a problem.

CASE REVIEW

Fatima presented with two very common conditions in pregnancy: back pain and anaemia. Both of these resulted in complex management plans and her antenatal care involved several different health care professionals. This case highlights the importance of patient handheld notes where each professional can record information in the same place. More details about routine antenatal care can be found in the Appendix.

Lumbar back pain is a common complaint in pregnancy, with up to three-quarters of all women affected (Brynhildsen *et al.* 1998). The symptoms experienced by women should not be trivialized. In the study by Brynhildsen *et al.* (1998), 19% of the women questioned who had low back pain in a previous pregnancy refrained from a future pregnancy because of fear of the severity of their symptoms. This study also demonstrated that unfortunately, in almost all women, symptoms returned in further pregnancies, as well as in the non-pregnant state.

The psychological components contributing to back pain can be complex and should always be explored with a patient as these can be important factors in determining prognosis. In this case, Fatima has several things that may be contributing including the stress at home.

Worldwide, the most common cause of anaemia in pregnancy is iron deficiency.

Although it is important to explore the patient's diet, low iron stores are most commonly treated by oral iron therapy. There are several different forms of oral iron including ferrous sulphate and ferrous fumarate.

KEY POINTS

- Up to 75% of pregnant women have lumbar back pain but it can be very severe in some, making them reluctant to conceive in the future
- Psychological problems can contribute to low back pain and can prevent it getting better
- Reassurance, paracetamol, physiotherapy, massage therapy and alternative therapies are all possible treatment options for back pain in pregnancy
- Worldwide, the most common cause of anaemia in pregnancy is iron deficiency
- Dietary sources of iron include meat, green vegetables (e.g. broccoli and spinach), cereals, strawberries and eggs
- Side-effects of iron supplementation include gastric irritation, nausea and altered bowel habit
- Side-effects can be reduced by taking the tablets with food or by reducing the dose

References

British National Formulary, 52nd edition. (2006) Royal Pharmaceutical Society of Great Britain. RPS Publishing and BMJ Publishing Group, London.

Brynhildsen, J., Hansson, A., Persson, A. & Hammar, M. (1998) Follow-up of patients with low back pain during pregnancy. *Obstetrics and Gynaecology* **91**, 182–186.

Fitzpatrick, M. (2003) Whiplash and other useful illnesses. *BMJ* **326**, 1092.

Garmel, S.H., Guzelian, G.A., D'Alton, J.G. & D'Alton, M.E. (1997) Lumbar disc disease in pregnancy. *Obestetrics and Gynaecology* **89**, 821–822.

National Collaborating Centre for Women's and Child's Health commissioned by National Institute for Health and Clinical Excellence. (2003) *Antenatal care: routine care for the healthy pregnant woman.* http://guidance. nice.org.uk/CG6 Accessed on 5 April 2007.

Case 28 A 42-year-old man with erectile dysfunction

Guy has been registered with your practice for 6 years. He is a handsome, slightly overweight man, tanned and wearing a good quality suit and striking tie. You have never seen him before, but you know his wife who is a parent governor with your partner at the local school.

He tells you with some bravado that he 'just can't do it like he used to' and his wife is worried about it. The nurse has seen him recently before for travel advice. He tells you that erectile dysfunction has never been a problem before. He wondered about getting some Viagra on the Internet to 'sort it out' but has heard that some of the tablets are a bit suspect and might be bad for your heart. He thought he had better see you first as his father had a heart problem.

Guy works hard and plays hard. He works as senior manager with a large accountancy firm, and manages their East Asia overseas business. He is married, and has three school age children. He was a fitness enthusiast although has put quite a bit of weight on recently as he has had less time for exercise since promotion.

He hardly ever consults and was last seen 4 years ago when your colleague referred him for a vasectomy. He had a short course of β-blockers for panic attacks when his father-in-law had a heart attack and his last child was just a young baby.

You ask for more information about the problem.

Despite his bravado he looks tense and you notice he is shaking slightly.

What questions might you like to ask him?
Physical
• *Erections:* quality, time of day they occur, circumstances in which he can get aroused
• *Sexuality:* is he exclusively heterosexual, has he had any other sexual encounters besides his wife?
• *Libido:* what is his sex drive like and has it changed?

• *Previous problems:* has this happened before?
• *Other symptoms:* especially those of vascular disease
• Past illnesses
• Smoker?
• *Alcohol:* how much and how often?
• Medications

Psychological
• Explore his relationship with his wife
• Is he under stress at home or at work or any other kind?
• Is he depressed?

Guy tells you he has not had much sexual activity in recent months, with his busy family life and long hours. The problem started suddenly after a recent trip to the Far East when he had unprotected sex with a female prostitute after a drinking game with colleagues. He had no difficulty getting or maintaining an erection during this encounter. He has never had a homosexual relationship.

He tells you he thinks about sex now and again but cannot be bothered. This has been a problem for a while. He has morning erections and if he masturbates and he is able to reach orgasm this way. The erectile dysfunction problem seems to be only with his wife.

He thinks he had a short-lived episode similar to this 4 years ago after the birth of his last child. He had an uncomplicated vasectomy 4 years ago. He is otherwise well. He smokes cigars occasionally. He has been drinking a bit more than usual (20 units/week). He is not sure he is up to the new job. His father recently had a heart scare and he worries about his own risks. He has taken β-blockers for anxiety in the past but none recently.

He has no other symptoms that might point to organic disease such as buttock pain, calf pain (vascular disease), thirst, polyuria (diabetes), parasthesiae or muscle weakness (neurological problem). On further questioning, he reports some dysuria since this episode.

What other questions might you ask him?

• Has he had any penile discharge or testicular pain that might suggest infection?
• Has his wife complained of any symptoms?

Guy admits to anxiety about having contracted a sexually transmitted infection (STI) through unprotected sex and says he is unable to tell his wife, as his marriage is already under stress. He is avoiding sex as a result. He is not sleeping well. He is afraid his wife will find out. He has not had any symptoms suggestive of an STI.

What possible causes are there for Guy's erectile dysfunction?

Physical and psychological.

Are you in a position to formulate a differential diagnosis?

• *Stress/anxiety:* fear of failure/guilt
• Relationship problems
• *Physical:* overweight, risk of diabetes, risk of STI (although this will not cause erectile dysfunction)

You check his peripheral pulses and his neurological status in the lower limbs. You also check the genitals.

This examination is normal. His weight is 78 kg and body mass index (BMI) 26.5.

Investigations are not very likely to help you make a diagnosis. However, they might be useful as supporting evidence, especially for vascular disease given the family history of heart disease:
• Cholesterol and other 'lipids'
• Fasting blood sugar level
• First pass urine for *Chlamydia*
• Urine culture for urinary tract infection
• Urethral swabs (dry slide sample and in culture medium) for non-specific urethritis (NSU) and gonorrhoea
• Blood pressure
• Electrocardiograph (ECG) recording

If erectile dysfunction coexists with low libido then it might be worth checking testosterone levels to exclude a hormonal problem.

You explain to Guy that you need to arrange some blood tests and will see him again in 1 week. His blood pressure is slightly elevated at 146/94 mmHg and you tell him you will check this again at the next appointment.

You will also ask the practice nurse to book him in for an ECG.

Guy is relieved that you are taking the problem seriously and not expressing any judgement about his extra-marital encounter.

One week later

Guy's blood tests are all within the normal range though his blood pressure remains slightly raised at 148/94 mmHg. Tests for STIs are negative and there is no evidence of a urinary tract infection. The ECG is also normal with no signs of ischaemia.

Can you now arrive at a diagnosis?

An acute on chronic psychological problem is most likely in view of his previous history, his present marital difficulties and his recent sexual experience with a prostitute and the guilt and anxiety that followed.

What is your management strategy?

• Deal with underlying worry: encourage him to tell his wife
• Discuss the problem of erectile dysfunction and how it is caused. Explanation and reassurance may help resolve the problem
• Acknowledge the psychological impact of erectile dysfunction on both parties. Suggest brief psychosexual interventions. This couple may need marital counselling
• Explore with Guy whether he is depressed. It may help to discuss lifestyle issues with him (e.g. workload, weight, smoking, drinking), and to discuss his concerns about heart disease
• Arrange review including another blood pressure measurement
• You might consider using medication in the short term but sildenafil (Viagra) and tadalafil (Cialis) are only available on private prescription unless there is an established physical cause for the erectile dysfunction such as diabetes or neurological damage. Referral to an urologist should be considered for consideration of other treatments if the problem persists.

Outcome. Guy refuses to tell his wife about his sexual encounter. You suggest psychosexual counselling and he reluctantly agrees to discuss this with his wife, but does admit he needs help with stress reduction.

PART 2: CASES

CASE REVIEW

Erectile dysfunction is common and can cause great distress (Tomlinson & Wright 2004). Patients now seek help and expect medical advice and intervention. While psychological causes and the effect of ageing are most common, other organic causes should always be considered. Vascular disease and diabetes are the most common physical causes for erectile dysfunction. Prostate surgery may also cause impotence. It is important to take a full and detailed sexual history as well as finding out about the quality of his erections, whether penetration can occur and orgasm. It can be difficult for both the patient and the doctor to discuss these issues so it is a good idea to have a few set questions that can be asked in a non-judgemental factual way.

In Guy's case, his libido is reduced but he has good erections, so his past history of β-blocker use and the vasectomy are unlikely to be relevant. This points to an acute on chronic psychological problem and an underlying relationship issue. It is important to deal with the possibility of an STI, as a negative test may resolve some of his anxiety. Some GP practices may not have the facilities or expertise to do penile swabs but a urine test for *Chlamydia* should be possible. Referral to a local genitourinary medicine clinic may be appropriate.

Guy does have some other features to be considered: cigar smoking, increasing alcohol intake and rising weight, but these are less likely to be the cause of his erectile dysfunction. They are important factors to be taken into account for future prevention of vascular disease.

KEY POINTS

- Erectile dysfunction is common and has considerable psychological impact on both partners. It should be taken seriously
- Physical causes including side-effects of medication should be dealt with. β-Blockers and many other medicines for high blood pressure can cause erectile dysfunction
- Drug treatment is helpful: unregulated Internet prescriptions may have implications for patient safety and interaction with prescribed drugs
- Other treatments should be selected and considered (Ralph & McNicholas 2000)
- Implications for prevention: care with β-blockers in men, early identification and careful treatment of diabetes; management of risk factors (for evidence for effects on libido see Rees & Patel 2006)
- In erectile dysfunction, the only modifiable risk factor is having a BMI of over 30 (Bandolier 2004)

References

Bandolier. (2004) www.jr2.ox.ac.uk/bandolier/booth/SexHlth/EDlife.html Accessed on 20 November 2007.

Ralph, D. & McNicholas, T. (2000) UK Management guidelines for erectile dysfunction. *BMJ* **321**, 499–503.

Rees, J. & Patel, B. (2006) Erectile dysfunction. *BMJ* **332**, 593.

Tomlinson, J. & Wright, D. (2004) Impact of erectile dysfunction and its subsequent treatment. *BMJ* **328**, 1037.

Case 29 A 64-year-old man with prostatism

Mr Abbott is booked into surgery. You know him well and feel you have a mutual understanding. He is a 64-year-old man who worked for the Royal Mail for 30 years, but is now retired. He spends most of his time on the golf course with his friends. You call him in, and he emerges from the waiting room and comes to see you. He tells you he is having trouble completing a round of golf because of the frequent need to pass water.

What questions would you like to ask?
- How long has it been going on for?
- Does it take time to start passing water?
- How often does he pass water at night?
- Any changes in the force of the stream?
- Ask about terminal dribbling
- Is it painful to pass water?
- Has he noticed any blood in his water?
- Has he ever been unable to pass water?

He tells you that his symptoms occur both during the day and at night. He tells you that he stands for some time before the stream is initiated. This has been a problem for him for 3 months. He has noticed the force of the stream is far less and there is significant terminal dribbling. He has not noticed any pain or blood when passing water and he has never been unable to pass water.

What likely problems are being described?
Lower urinary tract symptoms:
- Urinary tract infection
- Benign prostatic hyperplasia (BHP)
- Prostate cancer
- Bladder stones/cancer
- Neurogenic bladder

From the above, which are obstructive and irritative symptoms?
Obstructive symptoms:
- Hesitancy
- Poor stream

- Terminal dribbling
  Irritative symptoms:
- Urgency
- Nocturnal frequency

He tells you that he has heard about prostate problems, Nelson Mandela and Kojak have had prostate cancer and this is what he is mainly worried about.

What is the recommended primary care management of prostatism?
British Association of Urological Surgeons Recommendations for the Primary Care Management of Men with Lower Urinary Tract Symptoms (Speakman *et al.* 2004).

Recommended
- History
- Digital rectal examination
- Symptom score (e.g. International Prostate Symptom Score)
- Urinalysis

Optional
- Prostate specific antigen (PSA) test
- Urine flow rate
- Post void residual volume
- Frequency volume chart
- Urodynamics

What would you like to do next?
Abdominal examination and urine analysis.

The bladder is not palpable and groin lymph nodes are not present on abdominal examination. Urine dipstick negative for blood, protein, leucocytes and glucose.

How do you explain and obtain consent to perform a digital rectal examination?
You explain that it seem as though the problems are caused by an enlarged prostate and you need to examine

PART 2: CASES

Box 70 Chaperones

Wherever possible you should offer the patient the security of an impartial observer (a chaperone) during an intimate examination. This applies whether you are the same gender as the patient or not (GMC Guidance 2006)

---

him. This means that it is an examination 'from the bottom end' to assess the prostate size and surface (Box 70).

(As a female GP, I offered to perform the examination myself, to perform the examination with a chaperone or offered him an appointment with one of our male GP partners.) Mr Abbott chose to see Dr Andrews.

Two weeks later

He comes to see you 2 weeks later and says that he has seen Dr Andrews and has had the examination you suggested. You look at the medical records and note the documented examination record of an enlarged, smooth, soft prostate.

What does the examination findings tell you about the prostate following a digital rectal examination?

See Fig. 10 and Box 71 (Jones *et al.* 2004, section 6.10).

You explain to the patient that his prostate is enlarged. This means that it is pressing on the bladder and the urethra. Prostates enlarge with age and due to hormones.

He asks how you know that it is not something nasty such as cancer making it bigger? You explain that from how it feels it is very likely to be prostate enlargement as prostate cancer feels different on examination. From this explanation it is clear he may need further reassurance.

What further options do you have?

You discuss the PSA test (Box 72). This is a guide to the size of the prostate which may help reassure that all is well but does not pick up all cancers. PSA can also be raised in other situations such as after exercise, following

---

Box 71 Digital rectal examination of the prostate

Symmetrical, firm, elastic	Normal
Normal and enlarged	Suspect benign prostatic hypertrophy (BPH)
Normal and tender	Suspect prostatitis
Irregular consistency or hard node	Suspect prostate carcinoma

---

Box 72 Guidance on PSA testing

A man having a PSA test should not have a urinary tract infection, ejaculated in the previous 48 h, exercised vigorously in past 48 h, had a prostate biopsy within 6 weeks or a digital rectal examination within 1 week (Prodigy Guidance).

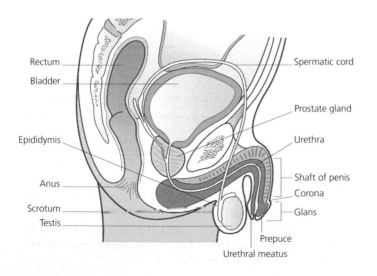

Rectum
Bladder
Epididymis
Anus
Scrotum
Testis
Spermatic cord
Prostate gland
Urethra
Shaft of penis
Corona
Glans
Prepuce
Urethral meatus

Figure 10 Male genitalia including scrotal contents.

prostate examination and water infection. Given the history and examination, if the result is low, the likelihood is that the prostate is enlarged as a result of BPH and not prostate cancer.

Following this discussion, Mr Abbott decides to think the options over and you offer a patient information leaflet about PSA testing (www.patient.co.uk/showdoc/23069165/).

Often, patients ask for a PSA test as part of a medical check-up. They may be of any age and may be asymptomatic. A similar discussion with those patients is useful.

On review 2 weeks later

Mr Abbott decided to take a PSA test (at the same time check renal function to help exclude renal impairment from possible long-standing obstruction). Some drugs will need dose adjustment in renal impairment (e.g. tolterodine and tamsulosin).

Mr Abbott's result is 3.2 (Table 9). You inform him that it is within the normal range for age and, given all the information, the likely diagnosis is BPH. You reiterate the options again: watch and wait or tablet treatment (Box 73).

He opts for treatment because the symptoms are such that he cannot even complete nine holes of golf and he is tired, mainly because of the night-time symptoms. In discussion with you, Mr Abbott chooses an α-blocker, because of his symptoms and preferred side-effect profile.

You prescribe tamsulosin MR 400 mcg/day, confirm he has understood dosing and side-effects and see him in 4 weeks.

Outcome. He comes back to see you and informs you that he has had no overt side-effects after the first week of treatment, and his symptoms have improved such that he can now complete 18 holes, just.

Table 9 Interpretation of prostate specific antigen (PSA) results (www.cancerscreening.nhs.uk/prostate/faqs.html#psa-test)

Age (years)	Normal PSA result (ng/mL)
50–59	<3
60–69	<4
70 and over	<5

> ### Box 73 Considerations for each treatment option
>
> **Watchful waiting**
> Education, monitoring, lifestyle advice (Speakman *et al.* 2004)
>
> **Lifestyle advice**
> Reducing amount of caffeine consumed, double voiding, caution not to reduce fluid intake to below 1.5 L/day (Speakman *et al.* 2004)
>
> **Drug treatment**
> 5α-reductase inhibitors (e.g. finasteride) block the metabolism of testosterone and can reduce prostate size by 30%, giving symptomatic results in 3–6 months (Prodigy Guidance). Side-effects to discuss with the patient are impotence, decreased libido, ejaculation disorders, testicular pain, breast pain and enlargement, hypersensitivity reactions (*BNF* 2006).
>
> α-Blockers (e.g. doxazosin, tamsulosin) are used for men with moderate to severe lower urinary tract symptoms and takes on average 4–6 weeks to have symptomatic benefit (Prodigy Guidance). They are thought to relax smooth muscle increasing urinary flow rate and improvement in symptoms. The side-effects to be discussed with the patient are postural hypotension, drowsiness, headache and dry mouth. The full information leaflet should be given (*BNF* 2006).
>
> **Surgical treatment**
> Referral should be considered for persisting symptoms despite medical treatment and troublesome symptoms

References

British National Formulary 52. (2006) British Medical Association and Royal Pharmaceutical Society of Great Britain, London.

General Medical Council (GMC) . (November, 2006) *Maintaining boundaries.* www.gmc-uk.org/guidance/current/library/maintaining_boundaries.asp Accessed on July 2007.

Jones, R., Britten, N., Culpepper, L., Gass, D.A., Grol, R., Mant, D., *et al.* (2004) *Oxford Textbook of Primary Medical Care.* Oxford University Press, Oxford.

Patient Information Leaflet. PSA from www.patient.co.uk/showdoc/23069165/ Accessed on 7 May 2007.

Prodigy guidance: *Prostate benign hyperplasia.* www.cks.library.nhs.uk/prostate_benign_hyperplasia/in_depth Accessed 7 May 2007.

CASE REVIEW

- Mr Abbott's symptoms were hesitancy, poor stream, frequency and terminal dribbling. These are mainly obstructive symptoms
- Consider the possibility of drugs leading to symptoms
- Abdominal examination and urine analysis were unremarkable
- Digital rectal examination is an important part of the assessment
- Intimate examinations should be conducted in a considerate manner, by a person who the patient feels comfortable with and a chaperone offered
- When an examination is not urgent, giving information and time can allow patients to make an informed choice
- As you will be working as part of a primary health care team, using the abilities and skills of other team members can enhance the patient experience and maintain trust within the doctor–patient partnership
- GMC guidance on chaperones suggests that during an intimate examination patients should be offered the security of the presence of an impartial observer
- Maintaining his lifestyle and concern about cancer were Mr Abbott's priorities
- Patient concerns and symptoms are priorities when deciding upon the treatment choices
- BPH can effect 10–50% of men over 60 years (Jones *et al.* 2004)
- Many men do not seek treatment (Jones *et al.* 2004)
- Renal impairment is associated with 1–3% of BPH (Jones *et al.* 2004)
- PSA testing should not be routine. PSA is raised in prostate cancer, BPH, prostatitis, exercise and following sexual activity
- BPH is caused by proliferation of the periurethral areas of the prostate, which leads to obstructive symptoms (Jones *et al.* 2004)
- Prostate cancer arises from the periphery of the prostate gland and is largely asymptomatic (Jones *et al.* 2004)

Prostate Cancer Risk Management Questions and Answers. www.cancerscreening.nhs.uk/prostate/faqs.html#psa-test Accessed on 7 May 2007.

Speakman, M.J., Kirby, R.S., Joyce, A., Abrams, P. & Pocock, R. (2004) Guideline for the primary care management of male lower urinary tract symptoms. *BJU International* **93**, 985–990.

An 82-year-old man with a cough

Mr Agnew, an 82-year-old retired scaffolder comes to see you in the surgery complaining of a long-standing cough. He has very little on his past medical record apart from an episode of depression 5 years previously after his wife's death. He lives on his own and is very independent. He is not on any regular medications. A man of few words, tall and still muscular, he has clearly been used to years of hard physical work.

What are your initial thoughts about the possible diagnosis?
Upper respiratory tract
- Rhinitis
- Post upper respiratory tract infection

Lower respiratory tract
- Chest infection
- Chronic obstructive airways disease
- Asthma
- Lung cancer
- Tuberculosis

Cardiovascular
- Heart failure

Gastrointestinal
- Hiatus hernia

What further information is needed from the history?
- Nature and duration of cough (e.g. if dry or purulent, any blood or wheeze, whether it occurs mostly when lying down)
- Recent cold, nasal blockage or blocked sinuses
- Smoking history
- General health including appetite, digestion, weight, night sweats
- Associated shortness of breath and if so whether this occurs when lying down

Mr Agnew has not had a cold recently and has been feeling well. The cough has been particularly troublesome for the last month; it is a little phlegmy but never wheezy. He denies coughing up any blood. His appetite and weight have been stable and he has been smoking 20 cigarettes a day since he was 18. He sleeps well, has not noticed any night sweats and the cough does not bother him at night. He does get short of breath on climbing stairs and on walking the dog, and recently has stopped going to the pub in the evenings. He does not have any chest pain.

On examination, his fingers are nicotine-stained but not clubbed, he is not cyanosed or short of breath at rest, and you do not detect any obvious abnormality in his chest apart from generally reduced air entry. He tells you that if you just give him some antibiotics he will be right as rain in no time. You check his weight which is 7 kg less than it was 5 years previously, giving him a body mass index (BMI) of 23.

What investigations do you do on Mr Agnew and why?
- *Chest X-ray:* will show up tuberculosis (TB), malignancy, chest infection
- *Full blood count:* anaemia, polycythaemia
- *Erythrocyte sedimentation rate (ESR):* TB, malignancy
- *Spirometry:* the most likely diagnosis is chronic obstructive pulmonary disease (COPD) secondary to smoking (Box 74)

Box 74 Chronic obstructive pulmonary disease

NICE (2004)
Diagnosis of COPD includes some or all of these features:
- Breathlessness on exertion
- Daily cough
- Regular sputum production
- Current smoker (64 pack years)
- Weight loss
- Wheeze

You also ask him if he has tried to give up smoking and offer help with this. He laughs and says he is too old to stop smoking now. He politely agrees to think about making an appointment with the practice nurse for smoking cessation advice. You book him in to the practice nurse's flu injection clinic the following week. Finally, you prescribe a salbutamol inhaler, taking care to demonstrate how he should use it, and arrange to see Mr Agnew again in 2 weeks.

Results

Full blood count (FBC): Hb 10.7 g/L with no other abnormal features (normal range 13.5–17.5 g/L)

ESR: 55 mm/h (normal range 1–10 mm/h)

Spirometry: FEV_1 60%, FEV_1:FVC ratio 0.6 (normal range 0.7–0.9)

Interpretation of examination and results so far

The general clinical picture is of mild COPD, but the normocytic anaemia and raised ESR are suspicious of a coexistent malignancy.

Three days later a radiologist telephones to inform you that Mr Agnew's chest X-ray showed an irregular mass in the right upper lobe and malignancy cannot be excluded.

What is the next step?

You need to refer Mr Agnew urgently to the chest clinic on the '2 week suspected cancer' referral system which you complete, attaching a copy of his X-ray and blood results.

You need to see Mr Agnew to prepare him. You telephone him to arrange for him to come and see you to discuss his results.

What do you say to Mr Agnew?

Mr Agnew attends with his daughter, Mrs Burrell. His first words are 'Is it cancer, doctor? How long have I got?' You explain that at this stage it looks as though Mr Agnew could have lung cancer but this is not certain and that he will need further investigations, probably including a bronchoscopy. He should take one stage at a time. His treatment would be explained and discussed with him step by step and he would be able to decide which treatment to have. You ask Mr Agnew if there is anything he wants to ask at this stage? Mrs Burrell becomes very tearful and asks many questions but he remains silent. Just before they leave Mr Agnew says in a quiet voice that he wants to die at home.

You arrange an appointment for 2 weeks time and stress that they can leave a message for you at the surgery in the meantime if there is anything you can do to help.

Two weeks later Mr Agnew has been seen in the chest clinic and the diagnosis of advanced, inoperable, poorly differentiated adenocarcinoma of the lung has been made. A course of palliative radiotherapy and chemotherapy is planned.

How do you continue to support him and his family?
On going care

You review Mr Agnew regularly in the surgery to check on physical and psychological symptoms. You also make yourself available to give support on the telephone.

Emergency care

You explain to Mr Agnew and Mrs Burrell how to access emergency care when the surgery is closed, and fax information to the out of hours service about him. You check you have Mrs Burrell's contact details.

Benefits

You explain to Mrs Burrell how to claim Attendance Allowance under Special Rules for her father, and give her your completed copy of the form DS1500 while sending a copy to the Department of Social Security.

You sign a form which entitles him to use a disabled person's badge to enable him to park as near to the hospital entrance as possible.

Liaison with other team members

You offer to refer him to the Macmillan Home Care Team and explain their role.

You discuss Mr Agnew in a multidisciplinary team practice meeting so that all the doctors and the district nurses are aware of his condition.

Mr Agnew receives a course of radiotherapy but chemotherapy is abandoned after two treatments because he develops profound neutropenia and is considered too frail to benefit from further treatment. He is now housebound and is visited regularly by the palliative care team from the Macmillan Service and the district nurses.

What symptoms is Mr Agnew likely to experience?
Physical

- Pain, both visceral and bony
- Constipation

- Nausea
- Cachexia
- Difficulty breathing
- Side-effects from drugs
- Difficulty with washing and toileting

Psychological

- Depression
- Anxiety
- Stages in acceptance of dying (Kubler Ross *et al.* 1969)
  1 Denial
  2 Anger
  3 Bargaining
  4 Depression
  5 Acceptance

What is the GP's role?

In many parts of the country, particularly in inner city practice, the GP's role has changed in recent years from 'hands on care' to one of coordination (Box 75). The district nurses and palliative care team visit the patient regularly and liaise with the GP in the surgery.

Box 75 Role of the GP in palliative care

- Streamlining and coordination of care. Providing continuity of care as far as possible by acting as a point of contact for the patient and their family, the district nurses, palliative care team, other GPs, hospital out of hours colleagues
- Prescribing, liaising with the pharmacist when necessary

Mrs Burrell has moved in with her father in order to care for him. One morning she requests an emergency visit. Mr Agnew has stopped eating and drinking and has become very weak and short of breath. During the night he developed severe lower abdominal pain and is writhing about in pain.

How do you manage him?

- Identify the source of pain
- Assess breathing
- Ascertain why he has stopped eating and drinking

Mr Agnew is severely wasted and his eyes are shrunken. Altogether he has lost several stones in weight. He has been refusing food and fluids for the past 48 h; previously he had been eating small amounts supplemented by high calorie

drinks on prescription. He admits to a lot of pain in his left hip and has been taking extra liquid morphine because of this. He has not opened his bowels for a week and is increasingly short of breath. Becoming suddenly very agitated he said he wants to die.

You sit down on the bed and try to reassure him. His abdomen is bloated and on rectal examination it is clear that he needs an enema. You ask the district nurses to administer this. He tells them that he is very upset because he wants to see his younger daughter, from whom he has been estranged, before he dies.

How do you manage these symptoms?

- Treat constipation: he may need a combination of a stimulant, bulking agent and a faecal softener
- Improve pain control: consider non-steroidal anti-inflammatory drugs in addition to regular morphine slow release (MST) and 4-hourly oral morphine as required
- Treat respiratory distress from bronchial secretions with hyoscine
- Assess mood: would he benefit from an antidepressant?
- Communicate clearly with his daughter, especially regarding changes in medications
- Check to ensure Mrs Burrell has adequate support at home; if appropriate discuss possibility of admission to hospice
- Make sure you have support for yourself from your colleagues in what is a very distressing situation

You revisit 1 week later. Mr Agnew's younger daughter is there, and he seems very much calmer. His pain is now well controlled on a syringe-driven morphine pump and you have converted his oral medications to the parenteral route. He continues to express his wish to die in his own bed in his own home. He is sucking ice but not taking any fluids now. The following Monday you receive notification from the out of hours service that he died peacefully at home at the weekend. Both daughters were present.

Finally

- Complete the death certificate. You have seen the patient in the last 14 days and the death was expected, therefore it will not be queried by the coroner
- Meet the daughters to see if they have any immediate concerns about their father's illness and death, or are confused about any arrangements

• Mrs Burrell, the older daughter, is registered as a patient at the practice. Think of contacting her a week or two after the funeral to invite her to the surgery to find out how she is coping with the bereavement
• Inform all members of the practice team and the out of hours service that the patient has died

CASE REVIEW

Mr Agnew suffered from chronic bronchitis resulting from 64 pack years of smoking which eventually caused his lung cancer. Breaking the bad news to him and his daughter was emotionally difficult for the GP who nevertheless let himself be guided by empathy. The GP coordinated appropriate services and benefits to control Mr Agnew's symptoms and give him the best quality of life, communicating well with the patient's carer, Mrs Burrell. The GP had the skills to alleviate Mr Agnew's physical and psychological problems as he deteriorated. Mr Agnew could only accept death when he became reconciled with his estranged daughter. This and the good network of carers enabled him to die peacefully in his own home in accordance with his wish.

KEY POINTS

The GP has an important role after diagnosis to:
• Give practical and emotional support
• Communicate sensitively with the patient and their family
• Coordinate care by communicating with all parties involved in the care of the patient
• Strive towards continuity of care
• Have overall responsibility for prescribing
• Identify and control symptoms
• Follow-up bereaved relatives where appropriate

References

National Institute for Health and Clinical Excellence (NICE). (February, 2004) *Chronic obstructive pulmonary disease.* Clinical guideline No. 12. http://www.nice.org.uk.

Kubler Ross, E. *et al.* (1969) On death and dying. *JAMA* **10**, 174–179.

The Gold standards framework: a programme for Community Palliative Care. www.goldstandardsframework.nhs.uk.

A 44-year-old man who wants a 'check-up'

Mr Leslie is a 44-year-old quantity surveyor who has recently joined your practice. You have not met him before. When he enters the room, you notice he is overweight and has a florid complexion. His records from his previous GP have not arrived yet. Mr Leslie says he does not want to bother you, but he wonders if he can have a 'general check-up'. He tells you that his wife has also been urging him to 'go and see the doctor'.

A request for a 'general check-up' is quite common in general practice. What should you ask next to explore the situation more?

- Was there anything in particular he was worried about?
- Was there anything his wife was worried about?
- How is his general health (e.g. smoking, drinking, exercise)?
- Has he had any serious medical problems or operations in the past?

You sense that there is some underlying anxiety as Mr Leslie appears nervous and his hands are shaking a little. You reassure him that you are there to help and you wait to see how he responds.

Mr Leslie says he is worried about his stomach. He has been feeling nauseous on and off and getting bouts of diarrhoea in the mornings. This is difficult when he is at work as he is getting a reputation for always needing the toilet. He thinks otherwise his general health is okay. He does not smoke but admits he drinks 'a fair amount'. He knows he is overweight. He says he used to play tennis but gave this up after he ruptured an Achilles tendon 4 years ago. He has not had any serious medical conditions or operations (apart from repair of the Achilles tendon).

You ask again if his wife was concerned about anything in particular? Mr Leslie looks embarrassed and says that

she is worried about the amount of alcohol he is drinking. When encouraged to expand on this and estimate how much he drinks on a daily basis, Mr Leslie says he is getting through 'a few' glasses of wine and 2–3 double whiskies. When pushed, he admits that this might increase to a whole bottle of wine and half a bottle of spirits on some days. This means he is drinking at least 10–15 units/day alcohol. You remember that a safe limit for a man is 21 units/week.

You wonder if this is the real reason Mr Leslie has come to see you. What other screening questions should you ask?

- Time of day of first alcoholic drink
- Pattern of drinking
- Withdrawal symptoms (early morning shakes or nausea)

Mr Leslie admits that he usually has his first drink before going to work to 'steady myself'. He does not drink at the office but at lunchtime he goes to the pub and has 'a couple of glasses of wine' with his colleagues. He leaves work around 18.00 and then sometimes pops into the pub on his way home. He has already mentioned feeling nauseous in the mornings and recently, he has also noticed his heart racing and some sweating, both of which improve when he has his first drink.

He does not drive, having had his licence suspended for a year after he was found to be 'over the limit' 8 months ago.

You are already getting a picture of a man with serious alcohol dependency. What further screening questionnaire would be useful?

The CAGE (**c**ut-down, **a**nnoyed, **g**uilty, **e**ye opener) questionnaire which consists of four questions:

1 Have you ever felt you should cut down on your drinking?

2 Have people annoyed you by criticizing your drinking?
3 Have you ever felt bad or guilty about your drinking?
4 Have you ever had a drink first thing in the morning to steady your nerves or to get rid of a hangover?

You explain to Mr Leslie that you would like to ask him some standard questions as above. A score of 2 or above indicates there is an alcohol problem. He replies 'yes' to all of them and admits he has been drinking regularly for years (Box 76).

Box 76 What are considered 'at-risk' or 'hazardous' levels of alcohol consumption?

- Over 40 g (5 units) of pure alcohol per day for men
- Over 24 g (3 units) of pure alcohol per day for women
  One unit in the UK means a drink containing 8 g ethanol (e.g. half a pint of 3.5% beer or lager or one pub measure [25 mL] of spirits). A small glass (125 mL) of average strength wine (12%) contains 1.5 units. People tend to pour themselves larger quantities of alcohol than this when drinking at home.

By now, you think it is likely that Mr Leslie's symptoms of diarrhoea and nausea are related to his alcohol consumption, but you want to clarify the situation.

What else should you ask?
- Has he had any vomiting and if so, has he ever brought up fresh blood of 'coffee grounds' (which might indicate gastrointestinal bleeding from an ulcer or severe gastritis)?
- Has he ever passed black tarry stools (melaena secondary to bleeding in the gastrointestinal tract)?
- Has he passed blood in his motions?
- Has he lost any weight (this is unlikely given his appearance but malignancy should always be borne in mind)?
- Is he depressed (many people who abuse alcohol have an underlying mental health problem)?

Mr Leslie has vomited occasionally after a heavy drinking session. He has never brought up blood or brown vomit to his knowledge and he has not had melaena. The diarrhoea tends to be during the mornings and then settle as the day goes on. He has not lost weight. In fact, his weight has steadily increased over the last few years.

He denies feeling depressed but admits that he has always suffered from anxiety and drinking helps him feel more relaxed and confident.

You ask Mr Leslie if he thinks his drinking is causing any difficulties, in particular in his job or at home?
Prodigy guidance (2007).

Mr Leslie says he has not missed any whole days off work because 'I'm not like that', but in the last few months he has been late for work occasionally, or not gone back after lunch if he has been at the pub. Because he can no longer drive, he is dependent on his work colleagues to take him to any jobs outside of the office and this is humiliating for him.

He admits that his wife has threatened to leave him if he does not stop drinking. At this point, he looks upset and stares at the floor. You reassure him that he was quite right to come to see you and you would now like to do a physical examination.

If he has liver disease secondary to alcohol, what might your findings be?
- Palmar erythema
- Spider naevi on the arms, neck or chest
- An enlarged liver
- Ascites
- Tremor
- Jaundice
- Gynaecomastia

You also measure his pulse, blood pressure, listen to his heart and check his height and weight and waist circumference.

Blood pressure 164/98 mmHg
Pulse 92 beats/min regular
Heart sounds normal, apex beat not displaced
Height 182 cm
Weight 94 kg
BMI 28.4 (25–30 = overweight)
Waist circumference 110 cm (if over 102 cm suggests risk of insulin resistance and metabolic syndrome)

Mr Leslie has a fine tremor in both hands and mild palmar erythema. He does not have any spider naevi or jaundice. The liver edge is palpable when you examine his abdomen even without asking him to take a deep breath in, suggesting that it is enlarged. There is no evidence of ascites or gynaecomastia (although both can be difficult to assess in the overweight).

What will you say to Mr Leslie about your findings and any further investigations that you want to do?

You decide that being absolutely straightforward in a non-judgemental manner is the best policy. You tell Mr Leslie that your examination has confirmed that he has signs of liver disease and this will progress if he continues to drink alcohol. He may have an enlarged fatty liver which could recover if he stops drinking. However, he is at risk of developing alcoholic hepatitis and eventually cirrhosis (scarring) of the liver, which is irreversible. His blood pressure is slightly elevated and there are many other health risks caused by excessive alcohol such as cancer, heart disease and pancreatitis, which would be greatly reduced if he managed to stop.

In order to assess the situation better, you want to arrange some blood tests to check his kidney, liver function and blood count and see him again a week afterwards. Mr Leslie looks worried. You give him a moment to take in what you have told him.

You ask if he has ever planned to stop drinking and if there is any help you can offer, such as seeing him with his wife and/or putting him in touch with the local Alcoholics Anonymous (AA) group?

Mr Leslie thanks you for being honest. He knows he has been drinking too much, but says now he has been given the facts, he will 'cut down'. He will talk to his wife about an appointment for them both to see you. He dismisses the idea of going to an AA group and says it is 'not his thing'.

What blood tests will you arrange and why?

• *Full blood count:* macrocytosis is common with alcoholic liver disease
• *Liver function tests:* often a raised gamma glutamyl-transferase (GGT) and alanine aminotransferase (ALT) or aspartate aminotransferase (AST)
• *Urea and electrolytes:* to assess kidney function as his blood pressure is raised

Mr Leslie leaves to go and make an appointment with the practice nurse for the blood tests and says he will see you a week later.

10 days later

You receive a hospital discharge letter informing you that Mr Leslie was admitted for 3 days following a seizure, thought to be secondary to alcohol withdrawal. He has been prescribed an anticonvulsant, carbamazepine 200 mg t.i.d. and chlordiazepoxide 50 mg q.i.d. (a short-acting benzodiazepine) in a reducing dose over the next 10 days, thiamine 200 mg/day (to protect against encephalopathy) and referred to the local addictions unit. One of the receptionists also tells you that Mr Leslie's wife has telephoned requesting a medical certificate for her husband. You check Mr Leslie's blood test results which show:

Full blood count: Hb = 15.6 g/dL
Mean corpuscular volume (MCV) 110 fL (normal range 80–96 fL)
Liver function tests: GGT 198 IU/L (normal range 5–80 IU/L)
ALT 112 IU/L (normal range 5–60 IU/L)
AST 79 IU/L (normal range 5–43 IU/L)
Bilirubin 0.9 mg/day (normal range 0.2–1.5 mg/dL)
Urea and electrolytes: normal

GGT may be normal in 70% of people who drink excessively. The other results showing raised enzyme levels confirm damage to the liver cells, although not specific to damage caused by alcohol. There are also other causes of a raised MCV such as folate or B_{12} deficiency.

You telephone Mr Leslie at home to find out what happened. Mrs Leslie picks up the telephone and says her husband is 'very poorly'. Apparently Mr Leslie had gone to work on Tuesday and had a fit in the office. This has never happened before. After the admission, various tests were performed before he was sent home on some new medicines. You arrange to do a home visit to see how Mr Leslie is feeling.

What is the significance of Mr Leslie having had a fit?

Withdrawal fits are not uncommon in those who are heavily dependent on alcohol and who experience physical symptoms such as the shakes, anxiety and sweats after a period of abstinence, or who drink to avoid such symptoms. Mr Leslie had told you that he had some of these symptoms so, in retrospect, you should have counselled him to reduce his alcohol intake slowly over a period of weeks or months.

The home visit

Mr Leslie is lying on the couch in his lounge and looks grey and unwell. He says he has 'been through hell'. After seeing you last week, he decided to go 'cold turkey' and stop drinking. On Monday night, he had no alcohol at all and woke up feeling 'awful' and shaky, but went to work and the next thing he knew he woke up in hospital. He knows he had some sort of seizure and has been told he must take the tablets to stop any further fits. He asks you if he will have to take them forever?

How are you going to respond and should you apologize to him for not making it clear that he should not have stopped drinking abruptly?

You can reassure Mr Leslie that the tablets are a temporary measure to get him through this period of withdrawal from alcohol. You decide that you should be honest and you apologize for not having advised him clearly about reducing his drinking slowly. Mrs Leslie bursts into tears and asks if her husband will ever recover?

What are the chances that Mr Leslie will be able to stop drinking and make a full recovery?

This is a very difficult question to answer as it depends on Mr Leslie's motivation and will-power. As his GP, you have a crucial role in supporting him and his wife and liaising with the local addictions unit. It is not appropriate for you to manage his detoxification as Mr Leslie is at risk of serious health problems (delirium tremens, fits, Korsakoff's psychosis) and will need hospital inpatient supervision. You say that you will find out how soon he can be admitted for treatment. In the meantime, you give Mr Leslie a medical certificate for the next 2 weeks and ask him and his wife to make an appointment to see you next week. You also check his pulse and blood pressure. He still has a slight tachycardia (pulse 92 beats/min regular) but his blood pressure has come down to 148/90 mmHg.

Back at the surgery, you telephone the addictions unit who confirm that they will be seeing Mr Leslie as an outpatient in 2 days' time. There are no beds available to admit him at present but he will be put on the waiting list for detoxification. They will prescribe any medication he needs and will fax you a copy of these.

Outcome. Mr Leslie attends the addictions unit on the first occasion and you receive a letter confirming that he will be admitted in the next 2 months, as soon as a bed becomes available. His wife turns up on her own to see you in the following week and says her husband has started drinking again. He is still on 'sick leave' and will not be able to go back to work until he has been admitted for treatment.

You give her the contact details of the local AA group and agree to provide a medical certificate that will cover Mr Leslie for 3 months.

Eventually, Mr Leslie is admitted to the addictions unit and manages to stop drinking for 5 months. He is made redundant from his job.

You wait to see if he can remain abstinent and retain his marriage. You see him regularly to monitor his blood pressure, mental health and general progress.

CASE REVIEW

Abuse of alcohol is a growing problem in the UK and a major cause of morbidity and mortality. Alcohol consumption is associated with 20–30% of hospital admissions (Ashworth & Gerada 1997). Nationally, it is estimated that an average GP will have 5–10 alcoholic patients per 2000 population per year (Cartwright & Godless 2003).

Alcohol is absorbed from the gastrointestinal tract easily and the ethanol is oxidized to acetaldehyde and then to acetic acid by enzymes in the liver. It is finally broken down to CO_2 and water through the citric acid cycle. Oxidation takes place at a fixed rate and so when saturation is reached, acetaldehyde accumulates and escapes into the blood stream. Here, it exerts toxic effects by inhibiting mitochondria reactions and functions. Long-term alcohol abuse leads to damage to the gastrointestinal tract, the liver and brain tissue.

Mr Leslie has a serious case of alcohol dependency and many patients you see will not have reached this stage of damage. For non-dependent drinkers, brief intervention by the GP including giving information about the effects of alcohol and advice on reducing intake can achieve more than a 20% reduction in alcohol consumption among problem drinkers (Ashworth & Gerada 1997).

For patients in Mr Leslie's position, detoxification must be undertaken in hospital because of severe withdrawal symptoms including fits and hallucinations. About 5% of people with severe alcohol dependency experience delirium tremens when they stop drinking. This generally occurs 72–96 h after the last drink and is associated with fever, severe hypertension and tachycardia, delirium, drenching sweat and marked tremulousness. It is a medical emergency because death can occur as a result of head trauma, cardiovascular complications, infections, aspiration pneumonia or fluid and electrolyte abnormalities.

The availability of addiction and substance abuse units varies tremendously around the UK and most have long waiting lists for both outpatient and inpatient treatment. Detoxification is also available in the private sector and in some medical units in NHS hospitals.

Although Mr Leslie does not want to attend Alcoholics Anonymous, many people find the organization provides essential support and practical help (the 12-step programme) for both the alcoholic and their family.

KEY POINTS

- Safe weekly limits of alcohol are 14 units for women and 21 units for men
- Harmful drinking is classified in the International Classification of Diseases (ICD-10) as a pattern of drinking that causes damage to physical (e.g. liver damage) or mental health (e.g. episodes of depression secondary to heavy consumption of alcohol; SIGN 2003)
- Screening questionnaires such as CAGE can be a quick and useful tool to assess hazardous drinking in primary care
- Blood tests such as MCV and liver function tests have low specificity and sensitivity but can be useful in demonstrating liver damage to the patient (and in

monitoring recovery when alcohol consumption is reduced)
- Many physical problems can occur with excessive alcohol use including gastritis, cardiomyopathy, cancer of the liver, mouth and oesophagus, breast cancer, diabetes, brain damage, accidents and injuries
- Close liaison with the local alcohol or addictions unit is crucial in helping a patient obtain detoxification and remain abstinent
- Voluntary organizations and self-help groups such as AA can provide essential support and expertise for patients and their families

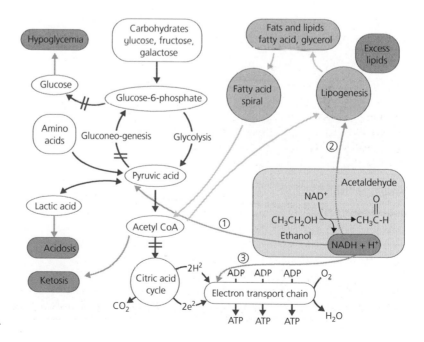

Figure 11 Metabolism of alcohol summary. Reproduced with kind permission from Dr Charles Ophardt, Professor of Chemistry, Elmhurst, IL, USA.

References

Ashworth, M. & Gerada, C. (1997) ABC of mental health addiction and dependence. II: Alcohol *BMJ* **315**, 358–360.

Cartwright, S. & Godlee, C. (2003) *Churchill's Pocketbook of General Practice*, 2nd edn. Churchill Livingstone, Edinburgh.

Metabolism of alcohol summary diagram. http://elmhurst.edu/-chm/vchembook/642alcoholmet.html Accessed on 14 November 2007.

Prodigy guidance. (2007) *Alcohol-problem drinking.* www.cks.library.nhs.uk/Alcohol_problem_drinking/ Indepth/Management_issues Accessed on 27 February 2008.

Scottish Intercollegiate Guidelines Network (SIGN). (2003) *The management of harmful drinking and alcohol dependence in primary care. A national clinical guideline.* http://www.sign.co.uk.

Voluntary organizations

Al-anon. www.al-anonuk.org.uk/
Alcoholics Anonymous. www.aa-uk.org.uk
Drinkline 0800 917 8282

A 49-year-old woman who feels exhausted

Nancy is a 49-year-old woman with two grown-up children. Her son, Simon, also appears in this book (Case 16). You have known Nancy for several years and saw her regularly when she was going through a stormy divorce, following which she was treated with antidepressants and psychotherapy. She runs her own oriental antiques business and often travels to India and the Far East. She comes to see you after a long time, complaining of exhaustion.

What are your initial thoughts?

• She might have been overdoing the travelling and have jet lag
• She is depressed again
• She might be starting to have menopausal symptoms
• She could have a viral illness caught on her travels, or a more chronic condition such as anaemia or hypothyroidism

What else do you need to find out to differentiate between these possibilities?

• Question about further symptoms to elicit a picture of her general health
• Find out how long the fatigue has been going on for and if Nancy thinks it was triggered by anything in particular
• Ask her about her periods, her sleep and any hot flushes
• Screen briefly for depression
• Elicit briefly the social context

This all may seem a challenge in a 10-minute consultation, which indeed it is. The art of general practice is to develop an effective and empathic way of consulting within the time constraints.

Nancy has no specific complaints other than feeling more and more exhausted over the last few months. She often goes to bed at 8 PM and wakes up in the morning feeling unrefreshed. She has missed one or two periods and when they come they are awfully heavy and draining. She has put on about half a stone because, she says, she no longer has the energy to do her daily yoga. This is beginning to get her down. She does not feel depressed, just 'Oh, so tired all the time.'

She has tried ginseng from the Chinese medical centre but this has not helped. She has been tending to be more constipated.

You are not sure if there are some underlying psychological issues, but overall you are beginning to suspect that Nancy might have a physical illness such as anaemia, hypothyroidism, systemic lupus erythematosus or chronic fatigue syndrome.

On examination, you do not find she is particularly pale, or that she looks floridly myxoedematous. She has no rashes and does not have a goitre. She is 5 kg heavier than when you last weighed her but that was 5 years previously. You have not checked her blood pressure for over a year so you do this and find that it is borderline and make a note to recheck it again next time.

What investigations would you do?

See Box 77.

> **Box 77 Screening blood tests for people who are tired all the time**
>
> • Full blood count
> • Erythrocyte sedimentation rate (this would be raised in systemic lupus erythematosus)
> • Thyroid function T4 and thyroid stimulating hormone
> • Autoantibody screen including thyroid autoantibodies and antinuclear autoantibody
> • You might also perform electrolytes and urea and liver function tests for the sake of a more complete blood screen

PART 2: CASES

Nancy asks you to add in a cholesterol test because her father died of a heart attack and she is trying to keep to a low fat diet.

Just as Nancy is about to leave, she says that she forgot to mention that she has been having pain and tingling in the thumb, index and middle fingers of both her hands during the night and sometimes during the day.

What is the likely diagnosis for these symptoms and how do you manage this?

Carpal tunnel syndrome. Wrist splints are likely to help more than anti-inflammatories. You write a quick note for her to take to the occupational therapy department so that they can supply her with splints.

You arrange to see Nancy next week to review the blood results.

Positive thyroid peroxidase autoantibodies
Raised thyroid stimulating hormone (TSH)
Low T4
Haemoglobin at the lower end of the normal range, full blood count otherwise normal
Cholesterol significantly raised

What is the likely diagnosis?

You make the diagnosis of Hashimoto's autoimmune thyroiditis. Nancy remembers that her mother has this condition too. She asks you, 'Do I have to stay on medication for ever?' (Box 78).

Box 78 Interpretation of thyroid function tests

- Primary hypothyroidism: raised TSH, low T4, usually positive autoantibodies
- Subclinical hypothyroidism: TSH slightly raised, T4 in the normal range. Monitor but do not treat unless patient has raised autoantibodies, thyroid enlargement or is symptomatic
- Low T4, normal TSH: indicates that the negative feedback loop is not working. Test for pituitary disease

---

How should you manage Nancy?

- Explain to her the nature of her illness
- Reassure her that she will feel better
- Emphasize that this may take several months
- Explain that she will need to be on medication for the rest of her life

- Inform her that she qualifies for free prescriptions of thyroxine and any other medication
- Start her on 25 μg thyroxine and arrange to check her thyroid function again in 6 weeks. Titrate by 25 μg 6-weekly until the TSH is in the normal range (Box 79)

Box 79 Titration of thyroxine

- Thyroxine can precipitate ischaemic heart disease, therefore it is safest to start with 25 μg in people over 40 years old and increase by 25 μg every 4–6 weeks
- Most people become euthyroid on 100–200 μg thyroxine. Rarely, some people require as much as 350 μg/day
- Aim to keep the TSH in the normal range
- If the TSH is suppressed, then the dose of thyroxine should be reduced, otherwise there is a risk of atrial fibrillation
- Thyroid autoantibodies can be monitored as a marker of recovery

---

After 4 months you are pleased to find that the thyroid function tests are normal with Nancy on 100 μg thyroxine. The autoantibodies are now negative. She is relieved to find that the cholesterol level is now satisfactory. Nancy is feeling a lot better but it takes a further 2 months for her to feel like her old self.

You insert a Mirena coil to control the heavy periods.

Six months after diagnosis she is feeling well. She had not noticed how dry her skin and hair had been, she is not constipated any longer and she has lost a few pounds.

Unfortunately, soon after this she comes down with a flu-like illness which she just cannot shake off.

What is your response?

- Recheck thyroid function
- Do full blood count, electrolytes and liver function tests to check for anaemia and other pathology

Nancy's thyroid function tests are very abnormal, with a grossly raised TSH and low T4. She also has abnormal liver function tests.

You are concerned and ring the duty endocrine registrar for advice. She tells you that the thyroid function is probably deranged because Nancy is getting over a viral illness, and that the thyroid should stabilize once she recovers.

She should have a 9 AM cortisol blood test to check that she is not developing Addison's disease.

Luckily, Nancy's 9 AM cortisol level is in the normal range and her liver function and thyroid function gradually return to normal as she recovers from the viral illness.

A few months later, having entered Nancy on your disease register for hypothyroidism, you review her notes. You can see from her prescription record that she must have run out of her thyroxine a couple of months ago. You telephone her and discover that she has spent the last few months at an ashram and ayurvedic medical centre in Bangalore practising yoga with a guru. She agrees to come for a review.

What do you say to Nancy?
• You ask her to explain why she stopped taking the thyroxine
• You try to address any concerns she has about her treatment
• You explain the importance of taking it regularly and having her blood monitored annually (Box 80)

Box 80 Difficulty in stabilizing thyroid function

• Can be a result of intercurrent illness
• Can be caused by compliance problems
 Some patients feel better if they take a higher dose than prescribed. This gives them more energy, keeps their weight down and suppresses TSH but it is not safe

---

The next time Nancy comes to see you, she shows you some information about Armour thyroid (dessicated porcine extract containing a combination of T4 and T3) which she has been buying from the Internet. She says she prefers to take this because it is more natural but would rather not have to pay to get it. What is your response?

Explain that you cannot prescribe this on the NHS and that it is not endorsed by the British Thyroid Society but it is probably safe so long as the patient is monitored and the TSH is kept in the normal range (Box 81).

Box 81 T3 and T4

Many patients believe that T3 (liothyronine sodium) is more effective than T4 (levothroxine sodium). Most T4 is converted into T3 in the blood, which is faster acting.
 At present, there is no firm evidence to say that T3 is more effective in the treatment of hypothyroidsm.

CASE REVIEW

Nancy is a middle-aged woman with a family history of Hashimoto's disease (autoimmune thyroiditis). She presented in a typically insidious way, and you were right to consider depression in the differential diagnosis, especially in the light of her past history.

As a consequence of her hypothyroid state, she also had carpal tunnel syndrome which resolved when she became euthyroid. Her raised cholesterol was also a consequence of her hypothyroidism and the level also came down to normal when she became euthyroid. The menorrhagia could also be related to the hypothyroidism or could have been caused by the peri-menopause.

Her thyroid function became deranged while she had a viral illness but returned to normal spontaneously when she recovered.

Nancy had some difficulties with accepting a chronic illness and the need to take medication for it indefinitely. Thanks to your disease register and recall system, you were able to follow her up actively. Nancy also had strongly held health beliefs which it was necessary for you to understand in order to treat her successfully.

KEY POINTS

• Non-specific presentation
• Often there are no obvious physical signs
• The dose of thyroxine needs to be titrated slowly until the TSH is in the normal range
• It may take several months before the patient feels completely better
• Once the condition has been diagnosed, it is important to put the patient on a disease register so that they can be recalled and monitored
• Many patients have strong health beliefs. It is often best to incorporate them in the management plan, provided this is safe

Case 33 A 62-year-old woman who is breathless

Mary is a retired teacher. She taught your children at school and is a keen walker, although sometimes she struggles to do this as much as she wants because she has osteoarthritis in her knees and hips. She only ever consults to have her blood pressure checked 6-monthly and this has been stable for several years.

It is a cold Thursday afternoon and you notice she is breathing heavily as she sits down in your room. She says she keeps feeling breathless. You notice Mary does not seem to have her normal sparkle and looks pale and tired.

What other information might you seek at this stage?
• Is she really short of breath or does she just feel breathless?
• How long has this been going on?
• How is it affecting her?

She thinks the breathlessness has been noticeable for a few weeks. It may have been a bit worse since a trip to Penzance on the train to see her only daughter, as she caught a cold and still has a slight cough. She found last week's walk with the rambling club too much and was unable to cope with the hills. She had to come home early.

What other questions might help?
• Did it come on suddenly or gradually?
• Is it worse when she lies down?
• Does she have a cough?
• Does she cough up any phlegm?
• Is the breathlessness worse at rest or on exercise?
• Does she get wheezy?
• Is there anything that brings it on (e.g. anxiety or panic)?
• Is there anything that tends to happens at the same time (e.g. nausea, palpitations)?
• Smoking history

• Alcohol consumption
• Allergies
• Occupational history
• Atopy
• Medications

Ask specifically about Red Flag symptoms that might indicate serious pathology
See Red flag symptoms.

> **!RED FLAG**
>
> • Weight loss
> • Haemoptysis
> • Sweats
> • Angina
> • Leg swelling

Mary says that the breathlessness has come on gradually over a few weeks and the cough is worse at night, but not the breathlessness. Recently, she brings up scanty yellow phlegm in the mornings. She is definitely more short of breath when she exerts herself, but this is not associated with any chest pain or wheeze. Mary is not aware of any allergies and she does not have eczema or hayfever. She has worked as a chemistry teacher in a secondary school for over 30 years.

She admits to smoking 40 cigarettes per day in her twenties, now less than 10 per day. She is taking a low dose β-blocker (propanolol 40 mg/day) for mild hypertension and anxiety. She does not have any of the Red flag symptoms listed.

She drinks no alcohol as she grew up with an alcoholic father who died prematurely of liver cirrhosis.

You decide Mary might have either a respiratory or cardiac problem, or be anaemic as she looks pale. There is nothing in her history to suggest a psychological cause or hyperventilation.

What common respiratory and cardiac problems can present with breathlessness?

Respiratory causes include:

• *Infection:* supported by cough with yellow sputum and smoking history

• *Bronchospasm:* smoking history, atopy, current β-blockers

• *Pulmonary embolism:* less likely, but should be considered in view of her recent travel

  Cardiac causes include:

• *Ischaemic heart disease:* often underdiagnosed

• *Arrhythmia:* such as atrial fibrillation

• *Mild heart failure*

  Breathlessness on exertion points to either bronchospasm or ischaemic heart disease.

  Mary has no history of allergy or atopy and she has been on the propranolol for several years.

When you examine her

Mary looks pale and tired. She is apyrexial.

Weight 75 kg, height 165 cm, body mass index (BMI) 27.5 (overweight)

Pulse rate 80 beats/min

Blood pressure 130/86 mmHg

Heart sounds normal

Peak flow rate 290 L/min (80% of predicted)

Chest examination: fine crackles at both bases

Jugular venous pulse (JVP) not elevated

No oedema or leg swelling

What further investigations might help you arrive at a diagnosis?

• Full blood count

• Urea and electrolytes

• Thyroid stimulating hormone (TSH)

• Brain natriuretic protein (BNP) levels (used to assess heart failure)

• Chest X-ray

• Electrocardigraph (ECG)

  You talk to Mary about your findings today and explain that you need to take some blood from her and ask the practice nurse to do an ECG this morning. You say you will also arrange an urgent chest X-ray. You ask if there is anyone who could take her up to the hospital for this?

  Mary looks very concerned. She asks if you can telephone her daughter in Penzance to explain what is going on. She has a friend with a car who might be able to go with her to the radiology department.

  You agree that you will talk to her daughter as soon as you have some more information from the investigations. You ask Mary to make an appointment to see you later that week.

Three days later

Haemoglobin 8.8 g/dL (normal range 11.5–16 g/dL)

Mean corpuscular volume (MCV) 76 fL (normal range 78–100 fL)

TSH normal

BNP 150 pmol/L – this is slightly raised. Levels over 220 pmol/L are more conclusive evidence of congestive heart failure

Urea and electrolytes normal

  From these results you can see that Mary has a microcytic anaemia. This is most commonly caused by iron deficiency. In younger woman, it is often a result of a combination of poor dietary intake of iron and heavy menstrual bleeding. In a postmenopausal woman such as Mary, blood loss for other reasons should be considered and also malignancy.

The ECG shows a sinus rhythm of 76/min and mild ischaemic changes with depressed T waves. The chest X-ray shows a slightly enlarged heart and some fine shadowing at the lung bases indicative of mild left ventricular failure.

What is your management strategy?

• Ask about diet, weight and blood loss (indigestion, vomiting and haematemesis, bowel habit, melaena [black tarry stools], haematuria or vaginal blood loss)

• Check what over-the-counter medication she might be taking

• Arrange investigation and treatment of anaemia

Mary says she eats a good diet, has not had any bowel symptoms or noticed any blood loss. She has had intermittent indigestion for a long time for which she takes Rennies (antacids). She has not had any vomiting. She would like to lose weight but has not been able to do so.

  Apart from the propranolol 40 mg o.d., she has been taking some naproxen (a non-steroidal anti-inflammatory drug; NSAID) for the last few months which her sister gave her and told her was good for joint pains. She is unsure of the dose but has been taking these for several months.

What examination and investigations should you arrange next?

• An abdominal and rectal examination to exclude obvious masses or rectal carcinoma. *You must offer to have a chaperone present to do this.*
• Arrange fasting lipids and blood sugar and iron studies
• Urgent referral to gastroenterology department for an endoscopy

What are you going to advise Mary?

You explain that the blood tests show that she is anaemic and this is probably caused by iron deficiency. You would like to examine her and then refer her to a specialist for further investigation and treatment. You suspect that the naproxen may have caused the problem and she should stop taking this and use paracetamol instead. You will prescribe her some iron tablets which will treat the anaemia while you are waiting for the outpatient appointment.

As the ECG and chest X-ray suggest she may have mild heart disease, you would like to check her cholesterol and blood sugar levels. You advise her that she would benefit from losing a little weight if possible.

You also ask her if she had thought about giving up or cutting down on her smoking.

Abdominal and rectal examination are normal with no masses palpable.

Mary agrees to see the practice nurse for smoking cessation and weight loss advice. She has been quite shaken by this experience and is more motivated to stop smoking than before.

You offer to speak to her daughter today, with Mary's permission, and discuss your findings. You arrange to see Mary again in 1 week and give her a prescription for the iron tablets. You tell her that she will have to take these for several months. You warn her about the common side-effects of taking iron (nausea, constipation or diarrhoea) and that she may notice her stools are black in colour while she is taking the tablets.

You counsel Mary against taking other people's medicines in the future, while acknowledging that her sister was only trying to help. You suggest she uses regular paracetamol, two tablets three or four times a day when her joint pains are bad.

Outcome. Further blood tests revealed low levels of iron and ferritin, which responded to treatment with ferrous sulphate 200 mg t.i.d. A repeat blood test after 2 months showed a haemoglobin of 10.2 g/dL and Mary was feeling much less breathless. A repeat chest X-ray after 1 month also showed clear lung fields and the heart was on the upper limits of normal size.

An endoscopy showed severe gastric erosions, thought to be secondary to the naproxen that Mary had taken. The gastroenterologist recommended an 8-week course of omeprazole 20 mg o.d.

Mary was found to have a raised total cholesterol of 6.0 mmol/L of which the high density lipoprotein (HDL) was 2.4 mmol/L. This gives a total cholesterol (TC): HDL ratio of 2.5. She was advised to go on a low fat diet and to stop smoking to lower her risk of ischaemic heart disease. She continued to have regular blood pressure checks and stayed on propranolol 40 mg o.d.

Mary's joint pains improved a little with paracetamol, but she said these were not as good for the pain as the naproxen.

CASE REVIEW

Breathlessness is a very common and important symptom, the cause of which is often multifactorial. This makes it a complex problem to sort out because cardiac, respiratory, haematological and psychological factors may all play a part. The prognosis depends on the predominant and most serious cause. Acute breathlessness often requires admission to hospital for further investigation and treatment.

In Mary's case, the breathlessness has come on over a few weeks and although she is obviously not well, she is not acutely ill, so there is time to arrange investigations and close follow-up at the surgery. Referral guidelines (Prodigy 2007) for suspected cancer recommend urgent referral to hospital for investigation of the gastrointestinal tract (upper or lower) if the haemoglobin is 10.00 g/dL or below. While malignancy is a possibility, particularly as Mary is a smoker, you have not found any signs or symptoms that make this high on the list of differential diagnoses.

There are several different reasons why Mary might be breathless. Anaemia is the primary cause and must be investigated and treated promptly. Breathlessness on exertion occurs because the oxygen-carrying capacity of the blood is reduced with lowered levels of haemoglobin. The respiration rate increases in an attempt to take up more oxygen. The anaemia is probably also contributing to her mild heart failure and there is a history of raised blood pressure which may be relevant. She is likely to have lung damage from smoking heavily as a young adult, although this was not evident on the chest X-ray.

Mary may also have residual infection from her recent cold and cough, exacerbated but being a smoker. However, as she is not pyrexial or particularly tachycardic, this is likely to be viral and require symptomatic treatment only. Iron deficiency anaemia can make people more prone to infections. There is no history of atopy so the breathlessness is unlikely to be due to bronchospasm from β-blockers.

Despite her recent long train journey from Penzance, there are no Red Flags for pulmonary embolism such as breathlessness in association with chest pain/dizziness or breathlessness with a unilateral swollen leg, so this is much less likely.

Mary has treated herself with a NSAID, naproxen. Although this is a prescription-only medicine which she got from her sister, several other NSAIDs are available over-the-counter. Adverse effects of NSAIDs are well documented and known to cause increasing morbidity and mortality with increasing age of the patient. According to one study (Blower *et al.* 1997), patients aged 45–64 years taking NSAIDs regularly have an annual risk of death of 1 in 3800 and of 1 in 646 of a gastrointestinal bleed. Some NSAIDs are more likely to cause adverse effects than others, with ibuprofen carrying the lowest risk and naproxen being more likely to cause problems. As mentioned in Case 14, NSAIDs can be combined with a gastroprotective agent such as misoprostol, but it is safer to advise patients to use regular paracetamol and topical NSAIDs for joint pains if possible.

Oral iron therapy should be continued for 3 months after the haemoglobin has stabilized to build up iron stores (Prodigy Guideline 2007). Iron is usually well tolerated but can cause indigestion, diarrhoea, constipation and nausea.

KEY POINTS

- Breathlessness is an important and common symptom
- It is often multifactorial
- Investigation of more than one cause is important
- NSAIDs carry a significant morbidity and mortality, mainly from adverse gastrointestinal effects
- Iron deficiency anaemia can lower immunity and make people more prone to minor infections
- Iron deficiency may be insidious as a result of slight blood loss over many months
- Haemoglobin levels would be expected to rise by 1.0 g/dL per month with oral iron therapy. It is usual to check the full blood count after 2–3 months of treatment and continue treatment for 3 months after stabilization of the haemoglobin

References

Bandolier Knowledge. *NSAIDs and adverse effects.* www.jr2.ox.ac.uk/bandolier/booth/painpg/nsae/nsae.html#Heading 10 Accessed on 1 December 2007.

Blower, A.L., Brooks, A., Fenn, G.C., Hills, A., Pearce, M.Y., Morant, S., *et al.* (1997) Emergency admissions for upper gastrointestinal disease and their relation to NSAID use. *Alimentary Pharmacological Therapy* **11**, 283–291 (quoted in Bandolier NSAIDs and adverse effects).

Prodigy guidance. (2007) *Anaemia – iron deficiency.* www.cks.library.nhs.uk/anaemia_iron_deficiency/in_summary Accessed on 3 December 2007.

Case 34 A 10-year-old girl with abdominal pain and recurrent vaginal discharge

Kelly is a 10-year-old girl with a long history of behavioural problems, soiling and enuresis. Different members of the primary health care team have seen her on multiple occasions, as her mother is concerned about her problems.

At home her mother looks after her and her 6-year-old sister. The girls' father sees both sisters regularly and has formal access to the children every other weekend.

Kelly's mother has brought her in today saying that she is having particular difficulty with controlling her at the moment. She says that her behaviour is often erratic and that school has recently been expressing increasing concerns about her lack of concentration in class and her disruption of others.

She has also brought her to see you a couple of times recently with vaginal discharge and genital irritation and apparently this has not settled with the treatment that you have given her.

What are the priorities during the consultation?

You need to listen carefully to the mother's concerns, finding out why she has brought Kelly today. You also need to clarify the history from Kelly and her mother.

What questions would you like to ask about her vaginal discharge?

• What symptoms is Kelly still having?
• Is there any discharge? What is it like? Is there any bleeding? Did the cream help at all (clotrimazole)?
• Does it hurt when she urinates?
• Do Kelly and her mother have any ideas about why the symptoms are not getting better?

Kelly is continuing to complain about itching and soreness 'down below' and the cream that she was given last time only helped for a couple of days. There is no burning when she passes urine.

Her mother thinks that she needs more treatment but is worried that Kelly's symptoms are because she cannot be bothered to wash herself and refuses help from her mother.

Which parts of the history particularly give rise to concern?

There are three areas of concern:

1 Ongoing enuresis and encopresis (faecal soiling) as these can have emotional causes
2 Vulvovaginitis that is resistant to treatment (Box 82)
3 Ongoing behavioural problems

> **Box 82 Differential diagnosis for vulvovaginitis**
>
> Royal College of Paediatricians and Child Health (2006):
> • Poor hygiene
> • Trauma
> • Skin disease including lichen sclerosis or eczema
> • Allergies particularly to soaps
> • Infection or infestation

What should you do next?

• Check that the previous treatment (clotrimazole cream for suspected thrush) was correctly administered
• Ask for any associated symptoms including abdominal pain, constipation and the impact of her enuresis and encopresis

Kelly says that she did use the cream that she was given but it did not help. Her mother adds that she has refused to go to school for a couple of days this week and that she has been complaining of tummy pain. She does not think that Kelly has had any bowel symptoms.

She has wet the bed most nights and also had wet pants a couple of times during the day during the last week. She gets upset and embarrassed on these occasions, particularly if she wets herself at school.

What would you like to do next?

It would be appropriate to examine Kelly now.

How would you ask to examine her?

You say that you want to feel Kelly's tummy and also need to take a look at her bottom to see why it is sore and itchy (just like you did last time she came). You ask both Kelly and her mother if this is all right.

Good practice would state that a chaperone should be present for the examination. You should also say that it should not hurt and that Kelly can tell you to stop at any time. You explain that you might need to take a swab and check her urine.

> They agree. Her tummy seems to be soft and non-tender with no positive findings. External genital examination confirms a red inflamed vulva but nil else of note. A low vaginal swab is taken. Urinalysis is negative.

What would be your management plan?

Kelly's symptoms and examination findings could have many causes but the most serious possible diagnosis is sexual abuse. With cases where it is not clear it can be extremely difficult to decide when a specialist referral needs to be made. However, the first principle is to minimize ongoing harm and so referral should not be delayed until the diagnosis is definite. This would usually take the form of a referral to a specialist paediatrician (Royal College of Paediatricians and Child Health 2006).

What further information would help with the diagnosis?

One line of revealing but non-threatening questioning could be to ask Kelly why she thinks the treatment has not worked. She may or may not disclose abuse and may be particularly reluctant to disclose anything in front of her mother. Remember that her answers may form part of the evidence for court and so extra care needs to be taken when recording the information.

You should also remember the importance of talking to other members of the primary health care team as you should not be working in isolation. They may be able to help you form a clearer history of Kelly and her family. It is also very important that you use your colleagues for support when having to deal with a case that is so upsetting (Fig. 12).

Which other agencies should be involved?

The Children's Social Care Department should also be involved early in the referral pathway.

Once you decide that specialist help is needed, how do you inform Kelly and her mother?

You tell them that you need to ask a specialist doctor to help with her symptoms, as you are unable to treat them on your own.

Would you tell Kelly or her mother of your specific concerns?

It is not necessary to share your concerns with the parents or the child, particularly if by doing so you may put the child at increased risk of harm. You should think carefully about disclosure before adequate discussions with your professional colleagues have taken place and protection achieved for the child (Royal College of Paediatricians and Child Health 2006).

Kelly's mother asks you if you think that there is something worrying going on. You respond by saying that you are referring her as you feel that you cannot properly treat her without specialist help. She tries to push you further on this but you are both interrupted by Kelly who says quietly that she would like to see the other doctor.

> Outcome. You call the paediatrician at the local hospital who deals with abuse cases. She agrees to see Kelly immediately at the hospital so that she can assess the situation. You are called to a case conference, to discuss Kelly, the following week. Kelly has disclosed that her uncle has been abusing her.

The immediate concern is for the safety of Kelly and her sister. They are not taken away from their mother as they are safe in her care while the police and courts ensure that the uncle cannot gain further access. Specialist teams along with the regular health care professionals further support the family.

> Kelly returns to school after the summer break with extra support from one-to-one teaching initially. She fully reintegrates after a term and her reports gradually improve. You have very little further contact with the family apart from dealing with the usual childhood illnesses.

PART 2: CASES

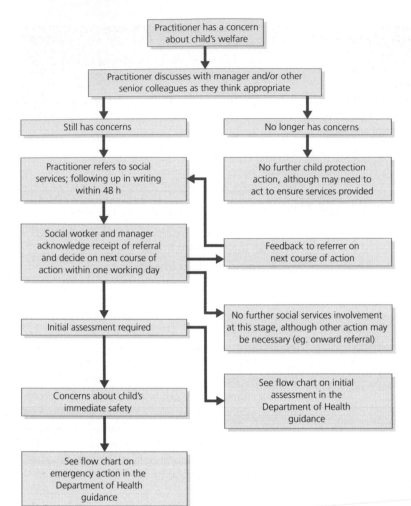

Figure 12 Immediate action. From Department of Health (2003)

CASE REVIEW

GPs hope that they will not have to deal with cases of child abuse but unfortunately its presentation is not infrequent. Abuse and neglect are forms of maltreatment – a person may abuse or neglect a child by inflicting harm, or by failing to act to prevent harm. The abuse may be physical, emotional or sexual.

All those who come into contact with children and families in their everyday work have a duty to safeguard and promote the welfare of children. It will lead to involvement in three ways (Department of Health 2003).

1 You may have concern about a child and refer to social services or the police

2 You may be approached by social services and asked to provide information about a child or family, be involved in an assessment or attend a child protection conference

3 You may be asked to carry out a specific type of assessment or provide help or service

It must be remembered that sexual abuse is often associated with other forms of abuse and that there are few absolutely diagnostic signs. The history taken should include a full urinary and bowel history, history of genital or anal symptoms, behavioral changes, menstrual and sexual history in adolescents (Royal College of Paediatricians and Child Health 2006). The use of specialists early on in the assessment is essential. If sexual abuse is strongly suspected then a paediatric forensic examination should be carried out by a specialist paediatrician and a forensic physician who will conduct a joint examination. This will involve:

- History
- Examination
- Documentation
- Obtaining forensic samples

If sexual abuse is only part of the differential diagnosis, for instance in cases of recurrent vulvovaginitis as in this case, a careful history and examination can be carried out by any suitably qualified practitioner (Royal College of Paediatricians and Child Health 2004).

As with all other procedures, consent must be obtained prior to examination. A child over 16 years can consent. Those under this age who fully understand the procedure and its implications can also consent (Gillick competency). If they are unable to consent, the parent or guardian can give consent for them but the child can still refused to be examined. A child can only be examined without consent if they are in need of urgent medical treatment (Royal College of Paediatricians and Child Health 2006).

Doctors must share information on a need to know basis with other agencies. It should be remembered that children are entitled to the same rules of confidentiality as adults but that it should not be allowed to stand in the way of child protection (Royal College of Paediatricians and Child Health 2006).

KEY POINTS

- All those who come into contact with children and families in their everyday work have a duty to safeguard and promote the welfare of children
- Abuse and neglect are forms of maltreatment. The abuse may be physical, emotional or sexual
- If sexual abuse is strongly suspected then a paediatric forensic examination should be carried out by a specialist paediatrician and a forensic physician who will conduct a joint examination
- If sexual abuse is only part of the differential diagnosis, for instance in cases of recurrent vulvovaginitis as in this case, a careful history and examination can be carried out by any suitably qualified practitioner
- You should not be working in isolation
- Remember that siblings may also be at risk

References

Department of Health. (2003) *Children's Services Guidance. What to do if you are worried that a child is being abused.* Department of Health Publications, London. http://www.dh.gov.uk/en/Publicationsandstatistics/Lettersandcirculars/LocalAuthorityCirculars/AllLocalAuthority/DH_4003423 Accessed on 22 March 2007.

Royal College of Paediatricians and Child Health. (2006) *Child protection companion.* http://www.rcpch.ac.uk/Publications/Publications-list-by-title Accessed on 22 March 2007.

Royal College of Paediatrics and Child Health and the Association of Forensic Physicians. (2004) *Guidance on paediatric forensic examinations in relation to possible child sexual abuse.* http://www.rcpch.ac.uk/Publications/Publications-list-by-title Accessed on 22 March 2007.

A 26-year-old woman with lower abdominal pain

Mrs Mzumbe is a 26-year-old woman who is well known to the surgery because she has had three children, all normal deliveries. You are on duty when she telephones for advice about her lower abdominal pain The practice has a doctor-run triage system whereby the doctor decides whether the patient needs to be seen on that day, given a routine appointment with a doctor or nurse, or needs telephone advice. She tells you that the pain came on suddenly, waking her up during the night and is getting worse.

What questions are important in the history-taking?

• Questions about the pain: site, whether colicky or constant, any aggravating or relieving factors
• Any vomiting?
• Any diarrhoea?
• Any loss of appetite?
• When were the bowels last opened?
• Any fever?
• Could she be pregnant?
• Any other urinary or menstrual symptoms?

Abdominal pain is a very common symptom with a very broad range of conditions from the self-limiting to the life-threatening (Fig. 13). A thorough history is the most valuable tool for making a successful diagnosis.

The answers to these questions may differentiate between gastrointestinal problems, diseases of the urinary tract or gynaecological conditions. On the basis of this you will be able make a decision as to whether the patient needs to be seen urgently, routinely, or advised on the telephone.

Mrs Mzumbe sounds anxious and distressed on the phone which is most unlike her usual self, and says the pain started off in the middle of her tummy after she had taken the children to school yesterday morning, but she had tried to ignore it. It came and went all day yesterday, but it had become unbearable in the night when it moved down to

the lower right-hand side and has been constant ever since. She has not wanted to eat or drink anything since the pain started and she has vomited twice. She has not opened her bowels for 48 h but this is not unusual for her.

You decide you need to see her immediately to exclude acute appendicitis and you arrange a home visit.

What has made you suspect appendicitis?

• The pain came on suddenly and is getting worse
• It is quite severe because it woke her up at night
• The pain in the peri-umbilical area, was colicky in nature and appears to have moved to the right iliac fossa where it has been constant
• She has vomited
• She has not opened her bowels for 48 h
• She sounds ill

Appendicitis is the most common abdominal emergency. You are right to have a high index of suspicion (Box 83).

Box 83 Acute appendicitis

• A delayed diagnosis of appendicitis can be fatal due to rupture and peritonitis with a mortality of 5.1 per 1000
• More common in males by 1.4 : 1
• Occurs mostly in children and young adults between the age of 10–20 years
• Typically presents with generalized abdominal pain localizing in the right iliac fossa due to spread of the inflammation to the peritoneum

---

Although you are thinking in terms of possible appendicitis, gynaecological pathology, such as ectopic pregnancy, pelvic inflammatory disease and ovarian cysts is also possible. Before leaving the surgery you make sure you put a pregnancy test and urine testing sticks into your medical bag.

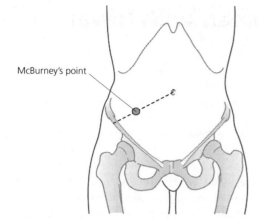

McBurney's point

Figure 13 Acute abdominal pain.McBurney's point represents a point of special tenderness in appendicitis, which is two-thirds of the way along an imaginary line drawn from the umbilicus to the right anterior superior iliac spine.

Mrs Mzumbe opens the door in her nightie. She is in tears, bending over and clutching her right lower abdomen. You take a history and then ask her for a urine sample while you clear the sofa of children's toys so that you can examine her.

What further questions do you need to ask?
- Has she had any pain on passing urine?
- When was her last period?
- Does she have any pain on sexual intercourse?
- Has she had any vaginal discharge?
- Has she had any history of pelvic infections?
- Any history of ectopic pregnancy?
- Has she had any vaginal bleeding?

She tells you that she has had some pain passing urine, that she cannot remember when her last period was, informs you that her husband uses condoms and that she does not remember having had any vaginal discharge. She has not had any ectopic pregnancies or infections or recent vaginal bleeding. She denies any pain during intercourse.

The pregnancy test is negative. The urine shows blood and leucocytes. You keep the sample to send off for culture and sensitivity. However, a urine infection is very unlikely to cause such acute symptoms.

You then explain to Mrs Mzumbe that you need to examine her. She looks very apprehensive and you are at pains to reassure her that you will be gentle and you explain what you are doing as you go along. You hope that talking to her in this way will also help her to relax her abdominal muscles.

What examinations will you do and what will you look for?
See Box 84.

Box 84 Examination of the patient with abdominal pain

General examination
- Patient's general condition: you have already decided she is ill as soon as you set eyes on her
- Pulse
- Blood pressure
- Temperature
- Oral fetor (bad breath)

Abdominal examination
- Note any scars and any distension
- Check the hernial orifices
- Palpate gently, starting furthest away from the pain then continuing to palpate the whole of the abdomen using slow pressure. Watch the patient's face to assess tenderness and observe any guarding
- Avoid testing for rebound as this is very painful for a patient with peritonism
- Use light percussion to test for maximal tenderness over McBurney's point which is two-thirds of the way along an imaginary line drawn from the umbilicus to the right anterior superior iliac spine
- Test for Rosvig's sign: positive if palpation of the left iliac fossa causes pain in the right iliac fossa
- Listen for bowel sounds to check peristalsis. It may take 2–3 min before bowels sounds are heard
- You may decide to do a rectal examination if the patient agrees, if you are still very uncertain about the diagnosis. On examination per rectum, test for pain in the right iliac fossa

Vaginal examination
- Explain to the patient why this is important and obtain her consent
- Test for cervical excitation and uterine or adnexal tenderness or enlargement
- You decide against taking a high vaginal swab and an endocervical swab for *Chlamydia* using a speculum. In any case this would be difficult in the patient's home where there is no proper lighting

---

Mrs Mzumbe is not so easy to examine as she is quite overweight. Bending over her on her sofa is giving you backache. She has a low-grade temperature of 37.5° with tachycardia. Her blood pressure is in the normal range. She is not flushed and has no oral fetor. The pain seems a little better on lying down. The abdominal examination reveals guarding in the right iliac fossa with an equivocal McBurney's sign. A few bowel sounds are heard. Vaginal examination reproduces pain in the right iliac fossa, there is no cervical excitation and no adnexal masses are felt which might suggest pelvic inflammatory disease.

What is your diagnosis and what do you do next?

You are not quite certain that Mrs Mzumbe has appendicitis but you think this is the most likely diagnosis.

Does she need any other investigations at this point?

See Box 85.

Box 85 Investigations in emergencies

- A plain abdominal X-ray will not help the diagnosis: this can be useful if you are looking for obstruction or stones but will not be diagnostic for appendicitis. Furthermore, you have decided that Mrs Mzumbe needs emergency admission in any case so it will not alter your management
- Computed tomography is the most accurate test for appendicitis in the hospital setting but is rarely used because of the urgency of the condition
- A vaginal ultrasound could reveal a cyst and this might be carried out in hospital prior to laparotomy
- A full blood count will not change your management either and would cause unnecessary delay
- You could have carried out swabs for *Chlamydia*, gonococcus and other sexually transmitted diseases, but this again would have caused more delay, and you are anxious to get the patient into hospital

---

You tell Mrs Mzumbe that she needs emergency admission. To your surprise she says she cannot possibly go into hospital and bursts into tears. She says she will be fine if you prescribe some strong painkillers and some antibiotics. You explain that you think she has acute appendicitis and that she needs an operation as soon as possible otherwise she could die of peritonitis if the appendix ruptures. She is panicking because she has no-one to look

after the children: her husband has had to go to Zimbabwe to visit his dying father. She pleads with you to delay admission until he comes back on Friday.

How do you resolve this problem?

Luckily the health visitor is in the surgery this morning. She knows Mrs Mzumbe well. You ask her to speak to the patient to see if there are any other friends or relations who could possibly look after her children in the short term.

Meanwhile, you return to the surgery to arrange admission, fax a referral letter to the surgical registrar on call and ask reception to call an ambulance.

The health visitor starts to liaise with Social Services so that the children can be taken into foster care. Luckily, one of Mrs Mzumbe's neighbours steps in to help so that the children can stay at home.

Outcome. Mrs Mzumbe had a laparotomy and was found to have a 6-cm simple ovarian cyst on the right ovary which was removed and sent for histology. The histology showed evidence of bleeding into the cyst but no malignancy. She also had her appendix removed which was found to be normal.

She made a full recovery, and only 6 months later you are congratulating her on her fourth pregnancy and arranging antenatal care for her.

CASE REVIEW

Mrs Mzumbe's symptoms were suggestive of appendicitis. Typical aspects of her presentation included the sudden acute onset of colicky pain moving to the right iliac fossa with guarding, her low-grade temperature and tachycardia. However, she had bowel sounds, no fetor and a possible urine infection.

An ectopic pregnancy was very unlikely as pregnancy tests are very sensitive. Moreover, as Mrs Mzumbe is a mother of three she would be likely to recognize the symptoms of early pregnancy.

It is not always possible to feel an ovarian cyst on vaginal examination. The absence of cervical excitation and uterine tenderness makes the diagnosis of pelvic inflammatory disease less likely.

You had to convince the patient that she needed admission for her own safety and your prompt and appropriate management was potentially life-saving.

KEY POINTS

- The GP has to work with probability and uncertainty. In primary care it is more important to recognize an acute illness and refer as an emergency than to reach a definitive diagnosis
- Appendicitis is the most common abdominal emergency in the UK
- The diagnosis of appendicitis is not always straightforward and must be considered from the history and examination

alone. The presentation and examination findings of an ovarian cyst and acute appendicitis can overlap. Definitive diagnosis can often only be made in theatre
- Other serious causes of right iliac fossa pain such as ectopic pregnancy should be considered
- It is important to consider the impact of the patient's illness on their family

---

Further reading

Humes, D.J. & Simpson, J. (2006) Acute appendicitis. *BMJ* **333**, 530–534.

Case 36 A 17-year-old girl requesting contraception

Melissa is a 17-year-old school student who is currently doing her A-levels. You have seen her occasionally over the last couple of years, mainly for troublesome acne and painful periods. There is no record in the notes of any serious illnesses or hospital admissions. She comes in today, looking a bit embarrassed and says she wants to go on 'the pill'.

As she seems very self-conscious, you reassure her that it is good that she has come in and thought about contraception. You say there are a few things you need to ask her.

What initial questions do you want to ask?

• Is she sexually active at the moment and if so, how long has she been having intercourse?

• What contraception is she using at the moment?

• Does she have a regular male partner?

• Has she had other partners in the past and if so, how long ago and were there any episodes of unprotected sex?

• Has she got any symptoms that might suggest a sexually transmitted infection such as vaginal discharge or discomfort on urinating?

• When was her last period and what is her usual pattern of bleeding?

Melissa says she has a regular 18-year-old boyfriend and they have been having sex for the last 6 months. She has had one previous partner over a year ago. She has always used condoms for contraception. She has not noticed any problems with discharge or dysuria. She is not sure if she has ever had unprotected sex, but if she did it was a long time ago. Her last period was 3 weeks ago and she usually bleeds for 6 days every 4–5 weeks.

This information gives you some idea of whether she is likely to be at risk of a sexually transmitted infection (STI) and/or pregnancy. From the information above, it seems unlikely she is pregnant or has an infection, but remember that some STIs such as *Chlamydia* may be symptomless.

In a 17-year-old girl with no previous serious medical problems, many of the contraindications in Box 86 would be highly unlikely. However, you should check whether Melissa has ever had migraines and if there is anyone in the immediate family who has had clots in the leg (deep vein thrombosis) or in the lung (pulmonary embolus) under the age of 45 years.

Melissa tells you that she does not have migraines. She thinks her mother's 52-year-old sister had a clot in the leg after being in hospital for a gallstone operation. No-one else in her family has had problems as far as she is aware.

Box 86 Absolute contraindications to the combined oral contraceptive pill

British National Formulary (2006):
• Focal migraine
• Liver disease, including infective hepatitis, adenoma, cholestatic jaundice
• History of venous or arterial thromboembolism
• Heart disease associated with pulmonary hypertension
• Uncontrolled high blood pressure (systolic >160 mmHg, diastolic >100 mmHg)
• Systemic lupus erythematosus
• Gall stones
• Past history of hydatidiform mole
• Breast or genital tract carcinoma
• Undiagnosed vaginal bleeding

Does this family history of thromboembolism preclude Melissa from taking the combined pill?

No. A family history of clotting disorders such as factor V Leiden or antiphospholipid antibodies which predispose individuals to thromboembolism would be significant, as would a spontaneous embolism in a first degree relative under the age of 45 years. A deep vein thrombosis after surgery is much more likely to be caused by immobility and/or obesity and should not affect your decision whether to prescribe the oral contraceptive pill or not (Prodigy 2007).

What other general questions might you ask Melissa?

- Does she smoke?
- Is she taking any regular over-the-counter medications?
- What is she using for her acne?
- Is there any family history of breast cancer?

Melissa tells you she does not smoke and she is not buying any over-the-counter medicines. She is taking minocycline 100 mg/day for her acne and has been on this for several months. It has helped improve her skin. Melissa is not aware of anyone in the family with breast cancer.

A strong family history of breast cancer (i.e. a relative under age 40, two relatives under the age of 60 or more than three of any age in the same family who have had cancer) might make you cautious about prescribing the combined pill to Melissa because this might suggest the *BRCA1* gene mutation. In such women, studies have shown that being on the combined oral contraceptive pill for more than 5 years increases the risk of early onset of breast cancer (Narod *et al.* 2002).

You ask her if she will remember to take the pill every day?

Melissa says she has managed to take the antibiotic regularly so she thinks she will be fine taking the pill every day.

It is always worth checking out whether the patient thinks she will remember to take a tablet daily. Some people are forgetful or lead disorganized lives which mitigate against remembering daily medication. In such individuals, you might consider the 3-monthly contraceptive injection Depo-Provera.

What examinations should you carry out?

- Weight
- Height
- Body mass index (BMI)
- Blood pressure (BP)

Should you offer to do swabs for a sexually transmitted infection?

You could do swabs as Melissa has had more than one partner and is not entirely sure whether she has had unprotected sex in the past. However, as she has no symptoms to suggest infection, you decide to concentrate on the contraceptive issue first and offer to take swabs at a later date.

Weight 62 kg
Height 1.65 m
BMI 22.8
BP 110/74 mmHg

These figures are all within normal limits. A woman who has a BMI over 30 is not recommended to go on the contraceptive pill because of the increased risk of thromboembolism.

What combined oral contraceptive pill are you going to choose?

There are many different brands of oral contraceptive available and it is a good idea to familiarize yourself with a few of these. You should also be aware of side-effects that might make one pill less suitable than another. It is common to start with a pill containing 30 μg ethinylestradiol combined with either 150 μg levonorgestrel or with 500μg–1 mg norethisterone. Examples of these would be Microgynon-30, Ovranette, Brevinor or Loestrin-30. These are all monophasic pills with a fixed amount of an oestrogen and progestogen in each tablet. Other preparations may be biphasic or triphasic with varying amounts of the two hormones according to the stage of the cycle. Examples would be TriNovum or Synphase (*BNF* 2006).

Melissa says she has heard of a pill that helps with acne as well as contraception and wonders if she can have this one?

Melissa is referring to Dianette, which has ethinylestradiol 35 μg and cyproterone acetate 2 mg. Cyproterone is an antiandrogen which probably decreases sebum secretion and so improves acne.

Would you consider giving Dianette to Melissa and if so, would she need to stay on the minocycline?

You could certainly discuss the options with her. The disadvantage of Dianette is that it contains a slightly higher dose (35 μg) ethinylestradiol than some other combined pills and it is not recommended for long-term use because of its antiandrogen effects. As Melissa has noticed some improvement in her acne with the minocycline already, she could remain on this and take a lower dose oral contraceptive at the same time which might also help her skin. The Dianette might be a second option after you see how she responds to a standard dose pill.

Melissa accepts this but thinks she might want Dianette in the future.

You decide to prescribe Microgynon-30 ED which has 21 active tablets and 7 white inactive sugar tablets. How are you going to explain to Melissa about taking the pill and when to start it?

You need to have a packet of Microgynon-30 ED (Plate 5, facing p. 56) on the desk so you can show Melissa what it looks like and which pill in the packet to start with. She could wait until the first day of her next period and then take a tablet on the corresponding day, starting in the dark strip on the packet. However, she may want to start taking the pill straight away today (also starting in the dark strip). If she does this, she will need to use condoms as well for 7 days, until the pill becomes effective for contraception.

Melissa is keen to start taking the pill before her period starts. This will mean her next period may be delayed until she starts taking the inactive sugar tablets.

What other information do you need to give her about the pill?

• The importance of taking the pill at the same time every day
• The 7-day rule for a missed pill
• What will happen while she is taking the sugar pills
• Things that might affect absorption and effectiveness of the pill

• Common side-effects
• Worrying symptoms that mean she stop taking the pill immediately (Box 87)

> ### Box 87 Reasons to stop taking the pill immediately
>
> *BNF* (2006):
> • Sudden severe chest pain
> • Sudden breathlessness
> • Unexplained pain in calf of one leg
> • Severe stomach pain
> • Serious neurological effects including unusual severe prolonged headache
> • Hepatitis, jaundice or liver enlargement
> • Blood pressure above 160 mmHg systolic and 100 mmHg diastolic
> • Prolonged immobility after surgery or leg injury

You explain to Melissa that the pill only works as a contraceptive if she takes it regularly at the same time every day. You suggest she might keep the packet with her toothbrush if she is good about brushing her teeth every night, as a reminder.

A missed pill may mean contraceptive cover is lost, especially if a pill is omitted at the beginning or end of the 21 days, so lengthening the pill-free interval. If Melissa misses a pill, she should take it as soon as she remembers it, and the next one should be taken at the normal time. If it is over 12 h since she should have taken the pill, she should use extra protection such as a condom, or abstain from sex for 7 days. If these 7 days run beyond the end of the packet, the next packet should be started at once, omitting the seven inactive tablets.

Melissa asks if she is still protected while she is taking the inactive sugar tablets?

While she is taking the inactive tablets, Melissa is still getting contraceptive cover provided she does not increase the length of time without an active tablet for more than 7 days. She is likely to have a withdrawal bleed for a few days during this time and it may be lighter and less painful than a normal period.

Reasons why the oral contraceptive might not work

Several medicines and over-the-counter remedies (e.g. St John's Wort) can make the pill less effective by interfering with its absorption. In particular, some antibiotics and various antiepileptic drugs can do this, and grapefruit juice. Because Melissa has been on minocycline 100 mg/day for several months, this will not affect the efficacy of the pill (see Case Review for further discussion), but if she is prescribed another antibiotic for anything, she should use extra precautions for the days she is taking this medicine *and* for 7 days afterwards.

She might not absorb the pill if she had an attack of diarrhoea and vomiting so you advise her about using other protection in these circumstances.

Melissa asks if she is likely to put on weight? She has a friend who went on the pill and put on 3 kg and she does not want this to happen to her.

You explain to Melissa that some women seem very sensitive to the hormones in the pill and do put on weight, but this is unusual on low dose preparations such as Microgynon-30. She may notice her breasts are tender and increase a little in size. Some women find the pill makes them nauseous, but this is less likely if she takes it at night. Other rarer side-effects are headache, mood changes, reduced libido, chloasma (increased pigmented patches on the face), high blood pressure and clots in the leg or lung. You can reassure Melissa that these worrying complications are extremely rare.

Melissa seems overwhelmed with all this information. You reassure her that you will give her some leaflets about the combined pill to take away with her and that she should look at the drug information leaflet inside the packet of pills too. The Family Planning Association leaflets (Family Planning Association, 50 Featherstone St, London ECY 8QU www.fpa.org.uk) on the combined pill (and other forms of contraception) are clearly written and contain information such as the 7-day rule and drug interactions.

How much oral contraceptive should you prescribe at this stage?
A 3-month prescription would be appropriate as you will want to see Melissa again at that time to recheck her blood pressure and weight and to find out if Microgynon-30 ED is suiting her.

What should you say to Melissa?
It is good to repeat some key messages. You suggest that she starts the pill straight away but remembers to use condoms for the next 7 days to ensure contraceptive cover. She should remember that the pill does not protect against sexually transmitted infections and for this reason she may want to go on using condoms anyway.

You do not expect her to experience any worrying side-effects, but if she is concerned or experiences any side-effects apart from the minor ones you have mentioned (breast tenderness and nausea), she should get in touch with you. You want to see her again *before* she runs out of the third packet of pills to check her weight and blood pressure again.

You ask if she is clear about the missed pill regime and using extra precautions for 7 days if necessary.

Melissa is able to reiterate the 7-day rule with your help. You give her the Family Planning leaflets about the pill and a prescription for Microgynon-30 ED.

Three months later
Melissa fails to turn up for a follow-up appointment and then comes in 6 weeks later saying that she has had to take the morning after pill and wants some more Microgynon-30 ED as soon as possible. She split up with her boyfriend and then had an episode of unprotected sex with a new partner.

What are you going to do next?
• Find out when her last period was and do a pregnancy test if appropriate
• Take triple swabs to check for STIs or suggest she attends the genitourinary clinic for these
• Make another appointment for Melissa when you have this information back so you can restart her on the combined pill (or discuss other contraceptives such as Depo-Provera), treat any infections and discuss 'safe sex' practices

CASE REVIEW

This is a fairly straightforward case of a sexually active teenager requesting oral contraception. The combined pill is appropriate given that she does not have any contraindications and its efficacy is still superior to the progesterone only pill or condoms alone (Table 10). Some antibiotics reduce the efficacy of combined oral contraceptives by impairing the bacterial flora responsible for recycling ethinylestradiol from the large bowel. If the antibacterial course exceeds 3 weeks, the bacterial flora develop antibacterial resistance and additional precautions become unnecessary (unless another
Continued

antibiotic is prescribed). If a woman has been on an antibacterial course for longer than 3 weeks and then starts the combined pill, as in Melissa's case, additional precautions are not necessary (except for the first 7 days if she starts the pill straight away and does not wait for her period).

Other combined pill preparations have not been discussed such as the third generation pills which contain gestodene. These are not recommended as first line therapy because of the slight increase in thromboembolic problems associated with them. They can be useful in women who experience side-effects with the progestogens norethisterone or levenogestrel and who have no contraindications such as a family history of thromboembolic disease, obesity or age over 35 years.

There is a lot of information to give to patients when prescribing the combined oral contraceptive pill for the first time and they are unlikely to remember everything. It is a good idea to give leaflets as well to back up your advice.

Many women stop taking the pill when they stop being sexually active for a time and do not anticipate needing it, as in Melissa's case. Advice about 'safe sex' using condoms and staying on the pill for several months may be appropriate.

KEY POINTS

- Combined oral contraceptives are reliable if taken regularly (0.08% failure rate; Bandolier 2007)
- Side-effects are usually minor
- The large number of different pills available with different combinations of oestrogen and progestogen mean a suitable preparation can usually be found for each individual
- Always advise the patient of the missed pill regime and 7-day rule
- Always advise the patient about concurrent use of other medicines or substances that might interfere with absorption of the pill and diarrhoea and vomiting
- Consider whether the patient is at risk of STIs – *Chlamydia* is often symptomless and its incidence is rising in the UK
- Advise about severe and uncommon side-effects of the pill
- Advantages of the pill also include reduced risk of ovarian and endometrial cancer

Table 10 Annual failure rates for contraceptive methods given both as a percentage failure in 1 year, and in the number of pregnancies per 10,000 women over 1 year. From BNF (2006) except combined oral contraceptive, calculated from Guilleband (2003).

Method	Failure rate (%)	Pregnancies per 10,000 women per year
None	85.00	8500
Cervical cap	30.00	3000
Sponge	30.00	3000
Spermicides	21.00	2100
Female condom	21.00	2100
Periodic abstinence	21.00	2100
Withdrawal	20.00	2000
Diaphragm	18.00	1800
Male condom	12.00	1200
Oral contraceptives	3.00	300
Progesterone-T IUD	2.00	200
Copper IUD	0.40	40
Injectable contraceptive	0.30	30
Tubal ligation	0.17	17
Combined oral contraceptive	0.08	8
Vasectomy	0.04	4

References

Bandolier. (2007) *Contraception: some numbers.* www.jr2. ox.ac.uk/bandolier/band50/b50-3.html Accessed 26 November 2007.

British National Formulary. (2006) British Medical Association and the Royal Pharmaceutical Association of Great Britain, London.

Guillebaud, J. (2003) *Contraception: Your Questions Answered,* 4th edn. Churchill Livingstone, Edinburgh.

Narod, S.A., Dubé, M.P., Klijn, J., Lubinski, J., Lynch, H.T., Ghadirian, P., *et al.* (2002) Oral contraceptives and the risk of breast cancer in *BRCA1* and *BRCA2* mutation carriers. *Journal of the National Cancer Institute* **94**, 1773–1779.

Prodigy Clinical Knowledge Summaries. (2007) *Contraception. UK Medical Eligibility Criteria (UKMEC)*. www.cks.library.nhs.uk/contraception/in_summary/scenario_combined_oral_contraceptive_coc Accessed on 4 December 2007.

MCQs

For each situation, choose the single option you feel is most correct.

1 *Which of the following is not a treatment for frozen shoulder?*

a. Acupuncture
b. Injection with intra-articular steroid
c. Manipulation under anaesthesia
d. Oral corticosteroids
e. Simple analgesia

2 *Which of the following is not a differential diagnosis for a patient with a sore throat and cervical lymphadenopathy?*

a. Bacterial pharyngitis
b. Gonorrhoea
c. Infectious mononucleosis
d. Thrush (pharyngeal)
e. Vocal cord polyp

3 *Which of the following is not an initial key question to ask a man with erectile dysfunction?*

a. Can he get an *erection* at any time?
b. Is his *libido* affected?
c. Is he taking any *medication*?
d. Can you talk to his *partner* about this problem?
e. What is his *sexuality*?

4 *What is the appropriate initial investigation for a 60-year-old smoker with breathlessness?*

a. Bronchoscopy
b. Chest X-ray

c. Full blood count (FBC), urea and electrolytes (U/E), thyroid stimulating hormone (TSH), chest X-ray, electrocardiogram (ECG), peak flow rate (PFR)
d. FBC, U/E, TSH only
e. Peak flow diary

5 *Which of the following is a test used to assess the knee?*

a. McMurray's test
b. Queckenstedt's test
c. Red pin test
d. Rinne's test
e. Rothera's test

6 *In herpes zoster which of the following dermatome infections always requires an urgent referral for specialist treatment?*

a. V1
b. C1
c. T1
d. L1
e. S1

7 *Which is the most appropriate antibiotic for suspected meningococcal septicaemia in a 27-year-old adult?*

a. Benzylpenicillin 0.2 g i.m.
b. Benzylpenicillin 1.2 g i.v.
c. Erythromycin 1 g i.v.
d. Rifampicin 600 mg i.v.
e. Rifampicin 600 mg p.o.

8 *Which of the following correctly states how blood pressure should be measured?*

a. Cuff 20% of the arm circumference, bladder placed over brachial artery with arm supported
b. Cuff 20% of the arm circumference, bladder placed over radial artery with arm supported
c. Cuff 40% of the arm circumference, bladder placed over brachial artery with arm supported
d. Cuff 40% of arm circumference, bladder placed over radial artery with arm supported
e. Cuff 40% of arm circumference, bladder placed over radial artery with arm unsupported

9 *Which is the most common sexually transmitted disease in the UK?*

a. *Chlamydia*
b. Gonorrhoea
c. HIV
d. Syphillis
e. *Trichomonas*

10 *Which of the following is true of prostate disease?*

a. There is a screening programme for prostate cancer in the UK
b. Most men with prostate cancer are diagnosed with it in their twenties
c. Prostate cancer is the most common cancer in men
d. Prostatitis is non-treatable inflammation of the prostate
e. Prostate disease commonly causes blood in the urine

11 *Which of the following is not used to assess the severity of asthma?*

a. Accessory muscle use
b. Amount of wheezing
c. Chest expansion
d. Pulse rate
e. Respiratory rate

12 *When should antibiotics be given in otitis media?*

a. If antibiotics have been given previously for otitis media
b. If deterioration occurs
c. If symptoms do not improve after 24 h
d. If the patient is aged over 2 years
e. If the patient swims regularly

13 *Lower respiratory tract infection is characterized by a cough accompanied by which of the following?*

a. Change in colour of sputum
b. Decreased chest expansion
c. Decreased sputum production
d. Sore throat
e. Wheeze

14 *NICE guidelines state that in the management of atrial fibrillation, rate control should be carried out in which of the following circumstances?*

a. Age under 65 years
b. No contraindications for antiarrythmic drugs
c. Presence of coronary heart disease
d. Rate >120 beats/min
e. Successful cardioversion

15 *Which of the following is not one of the differential diagnoses for irregular menstrual bleeding?*

a. Bleeding in pregnancy
b. Endometrial cancer
c. Menarche
d. Polycystic ovary syndrome
e. Vulval cancer

16 *In the treatment of panic disorder appropriate treatment could include:*

a. Electroconvulsive therapy (ECT)
b. Lithium
c. Long-term benzodiazepine use
d. Risperidone
e. Selective serotonin reuptake inhibitor

17 *In irritable bowel syndrome which one of the following statements is true?*

a. Typical features can include the following: diarrhoea, constipation, bloody stools, fever and bloating
b. It can be triggered by coeliac disease
c. It is prudent for patients to have regular colonoscopies because of the small risk of malignancy associated with the condition
d. It is a diagnosis of exclusion
e. Long-term low dose anticonvulsants can be helpful

18 *In depression which one of the following statements is true?*

a. Feelings of worthlessness or delusions of grandeur, weight gain or weight loss, hypersomnia and sleeplessness can all indicate clinical depression
b. Tricyclic antidepressants are safer in overdosage than the selective serotonin reuptake inhibitors (SSRIs) but have more side-effects
c. It usually takes up to a week before patients show any signs of improvement on antidepressants
d. Discontinuation syndrome can include the following: hypomania, panic, craving, nausea, vomiting and chills
e. Cognitive–behavioural therapy should be considered for people with severe depression, recurrent depression and people with mild depression who express a preference for psychological intervention over drug treatment

19 *In palliative care which one of the following statements is true?*

a. The Attendance Allowance under special rules (Form DS 1500) can be claimed if the patient has a prognosis of 6 months or less to live
b. In order to complete a death certificate, a doctor needs to have seen the patient less than 28 days prior to the patient's death
c. Non-steroidal anti-inflammatories are useful for neuropathic pain control
d. Morphine can be given by all of the following routes: oral in tablet and liquid form, transdermal, rectal, intramuscularly and by subcutaneous infusion

e. The stages of the grieving process in adjusting to death as described by Elizabeth Kübler Ross in her classic book *On Death and Dying* are as follows: denial, anger, bargaining and depression

20 *In primary hypothyroidism which one of the following statements is true?*

a. It is associated with tennis elbow
b. It is caused by autoimmunity, radioactive iodine treatment and pituitary tumours
c. Has a male to female ratio of 2 : 1 in the UK
d. It is associated with an increased risk of myocardial infarction
e. Can cause premature menopause in women

21 *In acute appendicitis which one of the following statements is true?*

a. It is the most common surgical emergency requiring operation in the UK
b. In pregnancy the management is conservative because of the risks of surgery to the fetus
c. Oral foetor, Kernig's sign, low grade fever and guarding are some typical signs of the condition
d. McBurney's point is two-thirds along an imaginary line drawn from the umbilicus to the middle of the right inguinal ligament
e. Typically starts with abdominal pain in the right iliac fossa followed by generalized abdominal pain increasing in intensity

22 *Which of the following is **not** true of hormone replacement therapy (HRT)?*

a. Breakthrough bleeding on continuous combined HRT is common but usually settles down after 6 months of therapy
b. Most women who choose to go on HRT use it for 1–3 years
c. Topical estrogens such as vaginal pessaries and creams will not relieve hot flushes
d. The risk of breast cancer is increased by HRT but remains low if it is used for less than 4 years
e. It is safe to give estrogen-only preparations to women who have had a hysterectomy

23 *In type 2 diabetes which of the following statements is correct?*

a. South Asians have a 10-fold increase in risk of developing diabetes compared to Europeans
b. Retinal screening should be carried out every 2 years to detect fundal changes such as microaneurysms and vessel proliferation
c. Aspirin 75 mg should be prescribed to all those with type 2 diabetes who have evidence of retinopathy or nephropathy
d. The Driving Licensing Vehicle Authority require all drivers who develop type 2 diabetes to inform the central office in Swansea
e. A diet based on 70% carbohydrate, 25% protein and 5% fat is suitable for someone with type 2 diabetes

24 *Select the most common cause for a 25-year-old patient with a red eye who has no relevant past medical history and is not on any medications, presenting in general practice*

a. Foreign body in the eye
b. Conjunctivitis
c. Keratitis
d. Glaucoma
e. Subconjunctival haemorrhage

25 *Which of the following statements about atopic eczema is incorrect?*

a. Emollients are the first line treatment for atopic eczema and should be applied four times a day if possible
b. *Staphylococcus epidermis* is the causative organism in most cases of infected eczema
c. Steroid creams should be prescribed for acute flare-ups of eczema in the lowest effective potency
d. Atopic eczema is common and affects 15–20% of school children
e. Infected eczema is evident by inflammation and crusting of the excoriated skin

26 *Which of the following statements is correct? Before a patient has a breath test or a stool antigen test for Helicobacter pylori they should:*

a. Stop taking any antacids such as Gaviscon for 1 week
b. Stop taking proton pump inhibitors (PPIs) such as omeprazole or lansoprazole for 1 week
c. Starve for 24 h before the test
d. Stop taking any antibiotics for 2 weeks before the test
e. Stop taking PPIs for 2 weeks

27 *Which one of the following statements is incorrect about stroke?*

a. Around 70% of strokes are thromboembolic and 19% haemorrhagic
b. Excessive alcohol consumption is a risk factor for stroke
c. Diltiazem and low dose aspirin are recommended as prophylactic treatment for anyone who has had a thromboembolic stroke
d. Half of all strokes occur in people over 70 years
e. Depression is common after a stroke and may be caused by organic brain changes

28 *Which of the following statements about alcohol is true?*

a. Alcohol consumption is related to 10–15% of hospital admissions
b. A small glass of average strength wine (125 mL) contains 1 unit of alcohol
c. A full blood count may reveal microcytosis in a patient who abuses alcohol
d. Screening questionnaires such as CAGE have limited use in primary care
e. An increase in the rate of breast cancer is seen in women who regularly drink over the recommended weekly intake of alcohol (14 units/week)

29 *Which of the following is not associated with bruising?*

a. Hypothyroidism
b. Thrombocytopaenia
c. Liver disease
d. Oral steroids
e. Factor V Leiden inheritance

PART 3: SELF-ASSESSMENT

30 *Which one of the following statements about termination of pregnancy is* **false**?

a. In 2004, 88% of NHS abortions were carried out at under 13 weeks' gestation

b. The risk of infection following a termination is around 10%

c. The 1967 Abortion Act allows termination of pregnancy before 24 weeks if it reduces the risk of mental or physical ill-health of the woman

d. Medical abortion using oral mifepristone, an antiprogesterone and a single dose of an oral prostaglandin can be used up to 9 weeks' gestation

e. Oral contraception following a termination should be delayed until the next period starts

EMQs

1 Urinary tract symptoms
a. Urinary tract infection (UTI)
b. Diabetes mellitus
c. Stress incontinence
d. Benign prostatic hypertrophy (BPH)
e. Urge incontinence
f. Haematuria

From the list above which is the most appropriate diagnosis?
1. Characterized by hesitancy, poor stream and terminal dribbling with a normal urine dipstick?
2. Characterized by urinary frequency, dysuria with nitrites and leucocytes on urine dipstick?
3. Characterized by leaking urine on coughing, sneezing and laughing with a normal urine dipstick?

2 Cardiac arrythmias
a. Ventricular fibrillation
b. Atrial fibrillation
c. Atrial flutter
d. Supraventricular tachycardia
e. Ventricular ectopics
f. Ventricular tachychardia

From the list above which is the most appropriate diagnosis?

1. Characterized by a sawtooth appearance on electrocardiogram (ECG)?
2. It appears as a narrow complex tachycardia on ECG?
3. It appears as a broad complex tachycardia on ECG?

3 Caring for people in their own home
a. District nurse
b. Health visitor
c. Home care
d. Occupational therapy
e. Chiropody
f. Community psychiatric nurse
g. Meals on wheels
h. Midwife
i. General practitioner

Which health care professional is described by each of the following statements?
1. Works under the umbrella of social services and can help patients wash and dress.
2. Works as part of the crisis resolution team.
3. Visits diabetic patients at home with poor mobility who are in need of foot care.
4. Visits patients at home and can perform many clinical assessments including falls.

4 Health promotion
a. Health education
b. Health protection
c. Precontemplation
d. Contemplation
e. Maintenance
f. Relapse
g. Health beliefs

Concerning the stages of change model of health promotion, which from the above list is the best fit for the following:

1. Suzie stopped smoking 6 months ago. Following stress at her workplace she has started smoking again.
2. George is a landlord at the Duck and Drake. He drinks 80 units of alcohol per week. He views his alcohol intake as not an issue as it is part of his job.
3. Wendy, a dinner lady, has painful knees. She has a body mass index (BMI) of 36. She has recently realized her weight is contributing to her knee joint pain and feels now is the time to do something about it.

5 Mental health
a. Anxiety
b. Panic disorder
c. Asthma
d. Depression
e. Obsessive compulsive disorder
f. Schizophrenia
g. Agoraphobia

From the list above, which is the most appropriate diagnosis?

1. Julia is 20 years old and finds she cannot leave the bathroom without washing her hands 18 times. She feels that if she does not do this she will make her mother and father ill by passing on germs.
2. Anne finds she frequently gets distressed, when her heart beats very fast, she gets sweaty and shaky and feels as if she cannot breathe and is going to die. There is no physical cause for her symptoms.
3. John is 43 and has recently lost his job. He feels worthless and has no self-esteem or confidence. He feels his future is hopeless. He has broken sleep and poor libido. He feels worse in the mornings.

6 Prostate examination
a. Normal sized, non-tender prostate
b. Enlarged smooth prostate
c. Irregular hard prostate
d. Enlarged tender prostate
e. Irregular small prostate

Which of the above findings on digital rectal examination corresponds best with?
1. Prostatitis
2. BPH
3. Prostate cancer

7 Management of hypertension
a. Angiotensin-converting enzyme (ACE) inhibitor
b. β-Blocker
c. Calcium channel blocker
d. Thiazide diuretic
e. Calcium channel blocker or thiazide
f. α-Blocker

According to the NICE management of hypertension of adults in primary care 2006:
1. Which is the first choice treatment for patients over 55 years or who are black?
2. Which is the first choice treatment for patients under 55 years?
3. Which is not currently recommended as a first line treatment?

8 Diagnosis of diabetes
a. Fasting blood sugar
b. Urine test for glucose
c. Glucose tolerance test (GTT)
d. Impaired glucose tolerance
e. Impaired fasting glucose
f. Diabetes mellitus
g. Normal glucose control
h. Random blood sugar

Which is the best fit from the list above:
1. It is the gold standard test for diagnosing type 2 diabetes?
2. Which are not diagnostic tests for diabetes in asymptomatic patients?

3. It is the diagnosis if the GTT result is
   7.8–11.1 mmol/L?

4. It is diagnosed if the fasting blood sugar is
   6.1–7 mmol/L?

9 **Treatment of type 2 diabetes**
a. Metformin
b. Gliclazide
c. Rosiglitazone
d. Diet and lifestyle changes
e. Insulin
f. Repaglinide
g. Acarbose

Which is the best fit from the list above:

1. Which is a sulphonylurea?
2. Which reduces peripheral insulin resitance?
3. Which is the first line treatment in type 2 diabetes?

1 *You get a call from the husband of a 59-year-old woman. He is requesting an urgent visit for his wife who is in bed with a severe headache. It started suddenly an hour ago while they were gardening. She thought that she had been hit on the head from behind by something but the husband cannot work out what it was. It is the worst headache she has ever experienced.*

a. Which of the symptoms are 'Red flags'?
b. What is the serious diagnosis that presents like a sudden blow to the head that must be ruled out?
c. What is the most appropriate management plan?

2 *A 42-year-old woman comes to the surgery during the first trimester of her third pregnancy. She had has a low haemoglobin (Hb) with each of her previous pregnancies. Her Hb has recently been measured as 10.2 g/dL.*

a. Should you worry about this?
b. What is the likely cause for her anaemia and how could this be checked?
c. What specific advice should you give her?
d. She asks you to remind her which foods contain iron. Name five.
e. Are there any other dietary substances that she should take or avoid?

3 *An 82-year-old lady is brought to see you by her daughter. Her mother moved in with her a few months ago and she has noticed that her mother sleeps a lot during the day.*

a. What are the possible causes?
b. You ask the mother if she thinks that there is a problem. She says that she has not slept well at night since the death of her husband last year and so she finds that she has no energy during the day. She has been feeling worse since she had to sell her home and move in with her daughter and her family. The information alerts you to the fact that she might have depression. What diagnostic tool could you use to formally assess her?
c. After a lengthy consultation with them both and after completion of the PHQ-9 you diagnose moderately severe depression. Are there any other tests that you would like to do at this stage?
d. Both of these tests come back as normal. What are your options for treatment?

4 *Arthur Smith was diagnosed with type 2 diabetes 11 months ago. He is an overweight 64-year-old and his treatment plan has included several oral medications to control his diabetes and reduce his cardiovascular risk.*

a. His annual diabetic review is now due. What should this include?
b. You see from the computer that he has not been requesting his medication regularly. What are the reasons for poor patient concordance?
c. He says that he is not sure why he needs to take all of the tablets and so you take time to explain each to him and supplement this with an information leaflet. You ask him if he knows what is a balanced diet for him. He asks you to explain it to him. What is a good balanced diet for a diabetic?

PART 3: SELF-ASSESSMENT

5 *A 72-year-old woman who is a known hypertensive and has osteoarthritis of the knees and hips attends the surgery for her annual blood tests. She is not diabetic and is an ex-smoker. She has a total cholesterol of 6.2 and high-density lipoprotein (HDL) of 0.8, blood pressure (BP) 138/88 mmHg at last reading; this means that she has an estimated 10-year cardiovascular risk of >20%. She is currently on two antihypertensives to control her blood pressure.*

a. What medications is she likely to be taking?
b. What are the annual blood tests that you would like to perform?
c. Are there any other tests that should also be carried out at her coronary heart disease medication review?
d. She says that she does not understand why she needs to take all of these tablets and admits that she often forgets to take some of them. What should you tell her?

6 *A 23-year-old telephone sales rep comes into the surgery asking you for antibiotics as she has had a sore throat and lost her voice for the last 2 days and is unable to work.*

a. What are the likely possible diagnoses?
b. You examine her and her throat is mildly red, her voice is hoarse and she has tender cervical lymphadenopathy. She has a temperature of 37.8°C. She wants you to take a throat swab as she has heard this will tell you what is wrong. Should you take a throat swab?
c. Would you treat this with antibiotics?
d. What are the sources of help that she could be advised to use next time?

7 *The physiotherapist at the local hospital contacts you as she has been seeing one of your patients with mechanical low back pain and it does not seem to be getting better despite intervention.*

a. What are the possible reasons for the patient not to respond to treatment?

b. What are the risk factors for chronicity of low back pain?
c. What is the name for the collection of alarm symptoms and signs for low back pain that would indicate that a serious disease has been missed? What are they?

8 *A 76-year-old man comes to the surgery with indigestion, tiredness and difficulty swallowing. It has been progressive over several months.*

a. What is the diagnosis that needs to be ruled out?
b. What could be the cause of his tiredness?
c. What are the other 'Red flag' symptoms and signs?
d. What should be the urgent investigation to confirm the diagnosis?

9 *A 5-year-old boy is brought to the surgery with a 'sprain' to his wrist. He is brought by his grandmother who says that this happened when he fell off the sofa. You examine him and he is very tender over his wrist and forearm, crying when you try to touch it.*

a. Should anything worry you about this?
b. What diagnosis needs to be ruled out?
c. What would be the most appropriate action plan?

10 *A 67-year-old woman attends the surgery with a cough. She is coughing up a lot more sputum and it is 'mucky' again. She thinks that she has another infection and it is the third one this winter. Her breathing is a bit worse than normal as she is having to stop twice on the stairs rather than her normal once.*

a. What is the most likely cause?
b. What is this secondary to?
c. What should you do?
d. No formal diagnosis has been made for her chronic breathing problems. What is the investigation of choice here?

MCQs Answers

1. d. The treatment is tailored to each phase of the disease. Acupuncture is a complementary therapy that could be used for this condition. Injection with steroid can be successful as it reduces the synovitis. Manipulation under anaesthesia is useful for refactory cases. Simple analgesia is often the mainstay of treatment in the initial painful frozen phase. Oral corticosteroids do not produce any lasting benefit and so should be avoided. *See Case 9.*

2. e. Although bacterial or viral tonsillitis and pharyngitis would be the most common diagnosis, alternatives include infectious mononucleosis and more rarely gonorrhoea or pharyngeal thrush. Patients with vocal cord polyp present with a hoarse voice and not a sore throat. *See Case 7.*

3. d. The following are the important questions to ask about in an initial assessment of erectile dysfunction: *erections, sexuality, libido, previous problems, other symptoms, past illnesses, smoking.* Although both partners should be treated, it is not appropriate to involve the partner in the diagnostic and investigative phase of the condition. *See Case 28.*

4. c. Shortness of breath can have many causes and so requires several different investigations at the outset. The differential diagnosis list includes lung disease including asthma, chronic obsructive airways disease, interstitial disease, lung cancer, pulmonary embolus, pneumonia; coronary artery disease; heart failure; heart arrythmia; panic attack; hiatus hernia.

   Although all of the tests above are used to diagnose a cause of shortness of breath, a broad net should be used initially and then further specialist investigations may be added depending on the initial results. Conditions can coexist and so several different tests should be performed. *See Case 33.*

5. a. McMurray's test is forced flexion with external rotation of the knee and it is used to test for meniscus damage. It involves placing one hand over the joint line of the knee and then flexing and extending the knee while rotating the ankle with the other hand. A 'click' may be felt over the joint line if there is a torn meniscus. Queckenstedt's test is used to detect a block in the circulation of the cerebrospinal fluid. Red pin test is used to outline the central visual field. Rinne's test compares hearing by air and bone conduction. Rothera's test is a chemical test for urinary ketones (Swash, M. 2007. *Hutchinson's Clinical Methods.* Saunders). *See Case 10.*

6. a. The herpes zoster infection can affect any dermatome. It can usually be treated in primary care, although it may become a medical emergency particularly if in an immunocompromised patient. Patients with any infection around the eye must always be referred urgently as it could lead to blindness. *See Case 11.*

7. b. Blind therapy for meningococcal septicaemia is benzylpenicillin given by intravenous or intramuscular injection at the dose of 1.2 g. *See Case 13.*

8. c. The guidelines state that the cuff must be of 40% of the arm circumference, the bladder must be positioned over the brachial artery with the arm supported. Additional guidance states that it should be measured in a temperate climate with the patient quiet. *See Case 18.*

9. a. *Chlamydia* is the most common sexually transmitted disease in the UK with 110,000 cases in 2005 and the number of cases is steadily rising. *See Case 24.*

10. c. There is no clear evidence that a UK screening for prostate cancer would be of benefit and so it has not been introduced. The risk of the disease increases with age and so it is diagnosed in older

PART 3: SELF-ASSESSMENT

men. It is the most common cancer in men, accounting for nearly one-quarter of all new male cancer diagnoses. It is the second most common cause of cancer-related deaths. Prostatitis is caused by inflammation but it is treatable; it can occur at any age. Prostate disease can cause blood in the urine but it is rare. *See Case 29.*

11. c. The severity is measured using the pulse rate, respiratory rate and degree of breathlessness, use of accessory muscles of respiration, amount of wheezing, degree of agitation and conscious level. Chest expansion correlates very poorly with degree of severity of asthma. It should be remembered that all the signs, used in isolation, can correlate poorly with the degree of airway obstruction. *See Case 2.*

12. b. Antibiotics should be given if deterioration occurs. They may also be given if symptoms do not improve after 72 h, if the patient is aged under 2 years or if the patient is immunocompromised. Whether they have been given previously should not influence whether they are given on this occasion. Swimming is a risk factor for otitis externa but should not influence antibiotic prescription in otitis media. *See Case 6.*

13. e. Lower respiratory infection is characterized by cough plus at least one of the following: increased sputum production, dyspnoea, wheeze, chest pain or discomfort, when symptoms have been present for under 21 days and there is no obvious alternative explanation for the symptoms. *See Case 1.*

14. c. Rate control for atrial fibrillation should be considered in patients aged over 65 years, those with coronary heart disease, contraindications to antiarrythmic drugs and those unsuitable for cardioversion. *See Case 19.*

15. e. Vulval cancer does not cause irregular menstrual bleeding. Irregular menstrual bleeding can be caused by pregnancy-related causes; anovulation which includes menarche, menopause, pituitary or hypothalamus problems, polycystic ovary syndrome, thyroid dysfunction; malignancy of the cervix or endometrium; infection. *See Case 25.*

16. e. In Case 21 the management of anxiety is discussed. The treatments used for panic disorder differ a little. Cognitive-behavioural therapy (CBT) and/or antidepressants are generally used. Long-term benzodiazepines should be avoided because of patient addiction and drug tolerance. Risperidone

is an antipsychotic agent and lithium is used in the treatment of mania, prophylaxis of bipolar disorder and in the prophylaxis or recurrent depression. *See Case 21.*

17. d. Bloody stools or fever would indicate inflammatory bowel disease. Irritable bowel syndrome can be triggered by an episode of gastroenteritis not coeliac disease. There is no association with malignancy but it is recommended to refer patients over 45 years old with new gastrointestinal symptoms to a specialist. Long-term low dose antidepressants rather than anticonvulsants can be helpful. *See Case 16.*

18. e. Delusions of grandeur occur in bipolar illness. False. SSRIs are safer in overdosage than tricyclic antidepressants and have fewer side-effects. When antidepressants are started it usually takes 2 weeks for the first signs of improvement to appear. Antidepressants are not addictive and do not cause craving when withdrawn. NICE guidelines confirm (e) is true. *See Case 22.*

19. a. When completing a death certificate a doctor needs to have seen the patient within 14 days of death. Non-steroidal anti-inflammatories are useful for bony pain and tricyclic antidepressants are useful for neuropathic pain. Morphine cannot be given by the transdermal route. The stages of the grieving process: the fifth stage, 'acceptance' has been omitted. *See Case 30.*

20. d. Primary hypothyroidism is associated with carpal tunnel syndrome not tennis elbow. Pituitary diseases cause secondary not primary hypothyroidism. It has a female to male ratio of 6:1 in the UK. It does not cause premature menopause. *See Case 32.*

21. a. In pregnancy surgical management may still be required. Kernig's sign indicates meningism. McBurney's point is two-thirds of the way along an imaginary line drawn from the umbilicus to the right anterior superior iliac spine. Typically, the pain is peri-umbilical to start with and then localizes in the right iliac fossa. *See Case 35.*

22. a. Breakthrough bleeding on continuous combined HRT is not common and should be investigated if it is present for 6 months as it may be a sign of genital malignancy (SIGN guidelines. www.sign.ac.uk/pdf/qre61/pdf). Most women use HRT for a relatively short time (i.e. 1–3 years). Topical estrogens will relieve urinary symptoms and vaginal

PART 3: SELF-ASSESSMENT

dryness but are not absorbed in sufficient quantities systemically to treat hot flushes. Data from the Women's Health Initiative Study (2002) suggested the risk of breast cancer was higher in women who took HRT for more than 4 years. In women with an endometrium, the risk of endometrial cancer is increased if unopposed estrogens are prescribed, but in women who have had a hysterectomy it is not necessary to prescribe a progestogen as well. *See Case 23.*

23. c. South Asians have a threefold increase in developing diabetes compared to Europeans. Retinal screening should be carried out annually to detect fundal changes. People with type 2 diabetes and retinopathy or nephropathy already have microvascular disease and are at higher risk of stroke and embolism. Aspirin is prescribed prophylactically because of its antithrombolytic properties.

   The DVLA does not require notification of type 2 diabetes if it is controlled by diet alone, unless relevant disabilities develop such as diabetic eye problems affecting visual acuity. A diet based on 55–60% carbohydrate, 15–20% protein and 20–30% fat is appropriate. *See Case 20.*

24. b. Unless the patient is in an occupation that exposes them to dust or other particles, foreign body is not as common as infection. Infective conjunctivitis (50% viral, 50% bacterial) accounts for about 35% of eye problems presenting in general practice (Royal College of General Practitioners and Royal College of Ophthalmologists 2001, quoted in Prodigy guidance). Keratitis is not uncommon but occurs less frequently than infective conjunctivitis. It is more common in people who wear contact lenses. Prevalence and incidence rates vary but NICE guidance estimates that 2% of people over 40 years and 10% of those over 75 years have chronic open angle glaucoma and so are vulnerable to acute glaucoma, but this is very unlikely in a person of 25 years old. Subconjunctival haemorrhage may occur spontaneously and may be brought about by raised blood pressure, clotting disorders or increased venous pressure (coughing). It is more common in the elderly. *See Case 5.*

25. b. *Staphylococcus aureus* and *Streptococcus pyogenes* are the two organisms most commonly associated with infected eczema.

Prodigy guidance suggests moisturization at least 3–4 times a day is essential to prevent dry skin and break the itch–scratch–itch cycle. Steroids can cause skin thinning and should be used for short periods at the lowest strength and stepped up or down in potency depending on the response to them. In the UK, atopic eczema is common but often improves as children mature. Crusting is pathogonomic of infection and should be treated with systemic antibiotics unless the skin involved is only a small area in which case topical antibiotics may be suitable. *See Case 12.*

26. e. Antacids can be taken continually. Proton pump inhibitors (PPIs) must be stopped for 2 weeks before testing for *H. pylori* because they can suppress the bacteria. No foods, liquids or smoking for 1 h before the breath test. Antibiotics must be stopped for 4 weeks before the test. A washout period of 2 weeks from PPIs is required to avoid a false negative result. *See Case 14.*

27. c. Around 70% of strokes are thromboembolic and 19% haemorrhagic, while a small proportion are a result of rare causes such as vasculitis, carotid artery dissection, a sudden fall in blood pressure or venous sinus thrombosis. Alcohol can cause vascular damage. Diltiazem is a calcium-channel blocker. It is a dipyridamole which is used with aspirin prophylactically because of their antiplatelet properties. Age is a risk factor for stroke. Depression is common and thought to be caused by a combination of circumstance and organic brain changes. *See Case 4.*

28. e. Alcohol consumption is related to 20–30% of hospital admissions. A small glass of average strength wine contains 1.5 units of alcohol. A full blood count is more likely to reveal macrocytosis but this test has low specificity and sensitivity. The CAGE questionnaire can be a very useful screening tool. Excessive alcohol consumption leads to an increase in risk of breast cancer and cancer of the mouth, oesophagus and liver. *See Case 31.*

29. b. Hypothyroidism can be associated with bruising. Thrombocytopenia (deficiency of platelets) is associated with bruising, thrombocytophilia would increase the risk of clots forming. Liver disease can lead to bruising because of deranged clotting factors. Oral steroids cause skin thinning which may lead to bruising. Factor V Leiden is an inherited disorder that increases the risk of clotting,

particularly if the individual is homozygous for the condition. *See Case 17.*

30. e. According to the Department of Health statistics, 60% of terminations were carried out at under 10 weeks. The Royal College of Obstetricians and Gynaecologists estimate an overall 10% risk of infection which may lead to infertility in the future. Reduction of the risk of mental or physical ill-health of the woman is the most common reason cited on the HSA1 form for a termination.

A single dose of mifepristone will induce abortion in early pregnancy but if medical abortion is used at later gestations, multiple doses of prostaglandin are required to induce labour. Oral contraception should be started immediately following a termination or miscarriage. *See Case 26.*

EMQs Answers

1
1. d
2. a
3. c

2
1. c
2. d
3. f

3
1. c
2. f
3. e
4. a

4
1. f
2. c
3. d

5
1. e
2. b
3. d

6
1. d
2. b
3. c

7
1. e
2. a
3. b

8
1. c
2. a, b, h
3. d
4. e

9
1. b
2. c
3. d

PART 3: SELF-ASSESSMENT

SAQs Answers

1

a. First and worst (single and sudden onset)
Sudden explosive headache (like a blow to the head)
b. A sudden explosive headache can indicate a subarachnoid haemorrhage
c. Visit the patient urgently:
  • Clarify the history
  • Examine the patient (vital signs, neurological examination: Glasgow Coma Score, opthalmological, cranial nerves, peripheral nervous system, extracranial structures: carotid arteries, sinuses, temporal arteries, cervical examination)
Arrange for urgent hospital admission.
See Case 3.

2

a. Yes, you do need to act on this. The normal range is defined as Hb >11 g/dL at booking or >10.5 g/dL in the third trimester. Very low Hb is associated with poor fetal outcome.
b. Although a drop in Hb during pregnancy is common because of haemodilution it could also be brought about by iron deficiency, particularly in view of her past history. It should be checked by a blood test to check her iron level.
c. As the level is outside the normal range you should discuss dietary intake, possible iron supplementation and follow-up.
d. • Meat
  • Green vegetables (e.g. broccoli and spinach)
  • Cereals
  • Strawberries
  • Eggs
e. Vitamin C helps the body absorb iron and is found in citrus fruits or cranberries including their juices. Tea and coffee reduce the absorption of iron and so should be avoided.
See Case 27.

3

a. • An organic disorder
  • Related to a depressive illness

• Patient and relative attending for another reason (e.g. relationship problems)
b. Commonly used scoring systems are the PHQ-9, Beck Depression Inventory and the Hospital Anxiety and Depression Scale. These should not be used in isolation but as an adjunct to clinical assessment.
c. Just because you have diagnosed her with depression does not mean that she does not have an organic disorder as well. You should do a full blood count (FBC) and thyroid function tests (TFTs) to rule out anaemia and hypothyroidism.
d. • Support
  • Bereavement counselling
  • Cognitive–behaviour therapy (CBT)
  • Antidepressants
See Case 22.

4

a. Assessment of:
  • Microvascular and macrovascular disease (inspection of feet, retina, urine testing for microalbinuria, blood pressure)
  • Blood tests (including measurement of HbA1c, renal function and cholesterol)
  • Medication review including patient concordance
  • Ongoing patient education including lifestyle changes
b. • Not knowing how to take the medication
  • Not understanding the importance of the medication
  • Taking several medications
  • Worries about anticipated or experienced side-effects
  • Forgetting
  • Impaired physical function
c. • Reducing fat
  • Increasing fruit and vegetable consumption
  • Increasing intake of fibre-rich starchy foods
  • Reducing salt intake
  • Increasing fish intake
  • Decreasing sugar intake
See Case 20; Case 11 for patient concordance.

5

a. • Aspirin
  • Statin
  • Thiazide-type diuretic
  • ACE inhibitor
  • Analgesics for her osteoarthritis
b. • Random blood sugar
  • Renal function
  • Liver function
  • Lipids
c. • Blood pressure check
  • Urine dipstick for protein
  • Check on patient concordance
d. You should inform her that although she does not feel unwell her raised blood pressure and high cholesterol mean she is at risk of a heart attack or stroke and that her medications are reducing that risk. You could give her details of her cardiovascular risk in specific numerical terms.
See Case 18.

6

a. • Viral pharyngitis/laryngitis
  • Bacterial tonsillitis/pharyngitis
  • Infectious mononucleosis
  • Pharyngeal thrush
  • Voice overuse
b. This has low sensitivity and specificity and so should only be used in persistent sore throat or treatment failures.
c. No, as the most likely diagnosis is viral laryngitis.
d. • Use advice from friends, family and past experience to manage the symptoms herself
  • Ask for advice from a pharmacist
  • Call for information from NHS Direct
  • Make an appointment to see the practice nurse or nurse practitioner
See Cases 6 and 7.

7

a. • Patient has developed chronic back pain after an acute back pain episode
  • Missed or alternative diagnosis and so treatment inappropriate
b. • Obesity, low education level, high levels of pain and disability
  • Distress, depressive mood, somatization
  • Job dissatisfaction
c. 'Red flags'
  • Weight loss, fever, night sweats
  • Nocturnal pain

• History of malignancy
• Acute onset in the elderly
• Constant or progressive pain
• Bilateral or alternating symptoms
• Neurological disturbance
• Sphincter disturbance
• Morning stiffness
• Immunosuppression
• Infection (current or recent)
• Claudication or signs of peripheral ischaemia
• Pain that is not improved with lying prone (with the stomach supported) or in the fetal position
See Case 8.

8

a. Upper gastrointestinal cancer.
b. He could be anaemic as the cancer could be causing some gastrointestinal bleeding and this can go unnoticed for some time.
c. Weight loss, vomiting and mass on palpation.
d. An urgent endoscopy should be arranged and also an FBC could be taken to assess whether he is anaemic.
See Case 14.

9

a. The mechanism of injury does not match the examination findings. In other words, it is a minor type of fall causing a bad sprain or possible fracture.
b. Non-accidental injury.
c. • To manage the injury appropriately including possible assessment in accident and emergency for an X-ray ± immobilization
  • To find out more information about the incident including any possible witness
  • To look in the patient's record to see if there is any previous concern about the welfare of the child
If you are still concerned about the child's welfare after hearing more about the incident, discuss with senior colleagues and ensure an appropriate referral to Social Services is made.
See Case 34.

10

a. Chronic obstructive pulmonary disease (COPD).
b. Smoking. Usually a patient will have smoked 64+ pack years.
c. Treat the infection. Re-educate the patient on the importance of stopping smoking and arrange for a follow-up to manage her ongoing symptoms.
d. Spirometry will show if she has COPD with a reduced FEV_1/FVC ratio, indicating an obstructive picture.
See Case 30.

PART 3: SELF-ASSESSMENT

Appendix: Additional information, schedules and normal values

The doctor's emergency bag

The GP's bag must be kept locked and not left unattended during home visits or on view in a car.

The following is a list of what could be carried:

- Stethoscope
- Sphygmomanometer
- Otoscope
- Tongue depressors
- Thermometer
- Pen torch
- Tourniquet
- Sterile gloves
- Reflex hammer
- Lubricant
- Tape measure
- Blood glucose monitor
- Peak flow meter
- Vaginal speculum
- Blood sample vials
- Syringes
- Needles
- Intravenous cannulae
- Urine dipsticks
- Water for injection
- Spacer
- Medication: benzylpenicillin injection, glyceryltrinitrate (GTN) spray, glucagon or glucose, epinephrine, bronchodilator, antihistamine, analgesic (oral and intramuscular), antiemetic, diuretic and hydrocortisone injection. It is essential that all drugs are checked at least twice a year to make sure they are still in date.
- Medical records
- Prescription pad
- Stationery
- Mobile telephone
- *British National Formulary*
- Local map

There is considerable debate about what should be carried. It depends on the regularity of visits, area of practice including important factors such as how far the patient is from secondary care.

A study from Belgium, the European leaders in home visits, in 2002 asked GPs what they carried and the list above has been partly created from this. Some items are used on more than one-third of all visits (e.g. stethoscope, sphygmanometer and prescription pad), others are required rarely but are carried for particular medical emergencies. GPs working in more isolated areas may carry an airway and oxygen cylinder, an automated external defibrillator and thrombolytic drugs.

Reference: Devroey, D., Cogge, M. & Betz, W. (2002) Do general practitioners use what is in their doctor's bag? *Scandinavian Journal of Primary Care* **20**, 242–243.

Estimated number of patients consulting a GP by selected disease/condition, UK, 2002

Disease/condition	Patients (000s)	Disease/condition	Patients (000s)
Infectious and parasitic diseases	5,496	Respiratory system	13,876
Neoplasms	1,500	Digestive system	6,476
Blood and blood-forming organs	651	Skin and subcutaneous tissue	9,775
Endocrine, nutritional and metabolic diseases	3,986	Musculoskeletal system and connective tissue	9,937
Mental and behavioural disorders	5,270	Genitourinary system	6,738
Nervous system	3,012	Pregnancy, childbirth and the puerperium	348
Eye and adnexa	4,025	Conditions of the perinatal period	59
Ear and mastoid process	4,007	Congenital anomalies	309
Circulatory system	8,047	Injury and poisoning	5,832

Reference: Office of Health Economics. (2003/2004) *Compendium of Health Statistics*, 15th edn. OHE, London.

Immunization schedule in the UK

The NHS immunization website gives comprehensive information about the reasons behind the vaccination programme, how they work and details about each vaccine used including the risks.

When to immunize	Diseases protected against	Vaccine given
2 months	Diptheria, tetanus, pertussis, polio, *Haemophilus influenza* type b, pneumococcal	DTaP/IPV/Hib + Pneumococcal conjugate vaccine (PCV)
3 months	Diptheria, tetanus, pertussis, polio, *Haemophilus influenza* type b, meningitis C	DTaP/IPV/Hib + Men C
4 months	Diptheria, tetanus, pertussis, polio, *Haemophilus influenza* type b, meningitis C, pneumococcal	DTaP/IPV/Hib + Men C + PCV
Around 12 months	*Haemophilus influenza* type b, meningitis C	Hib/Men C
Around 13 months	Measles, mumps, rubella, pneumococcal	MMR + PCV
3 years 4 months–5 years	Diptheria, tetanus, pertussis, polio, measles, mumps, rubella	DTaP/IPV/Hib or dTaP/IPV + MMR
13–18 years	Tetanus, diphtheria, polio	Td/IPV

Reference: http://www.immunisation.nhs.uk/article.php?id=55.

Normal respiratory and pulse rates in children

Age (years)	Respiratory rate (breaths/min)	Pulse rate (beats/min)
<1	30–40	110–160
1–2	25–35	100–150
2–5	25–30	95–140
5–12	20–25	80–120
>12	15–20	60–100

Reference: Joint Royal Colleges Ambulance Liaison Committee. (2004) *Recognition of the Seriously Ill Child*. Joint Royal Colleges Ambulance Liaison Committee, London.

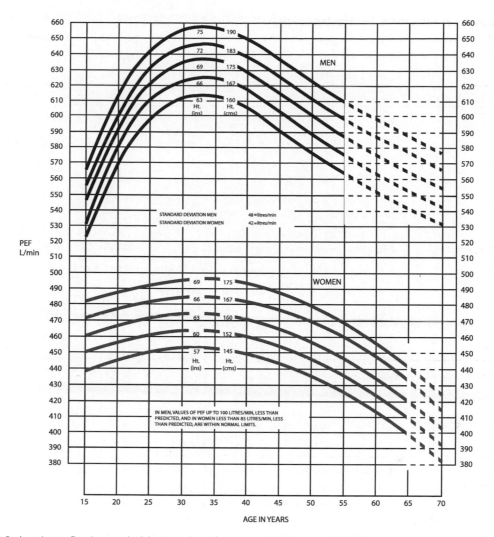

Figure 14 Peak expiratory flow in normal adults. Reproduced from Nunn, A.J. & Gregg, I. (1989) New regression equations for predicting peak expiratory flow in adults. *BMJ* **298**, 1068–1070, with permission from the BMJ Publishing Group.

Predicted normal values for spirometry

These values apply to Caucasians, reduce values by 7% for Asians and by 13% for Afro-Carribbeans.

Male

Age (years)		5′3″ 160 cm	5′5″ 165 cm	5′7″ 170 cm	5′9″ 180 cm	5′11″ 185 cm	6′1″ 190 cm	6′3″ 195 cm
38–41	FVC	3.81	4.20	4.39	4.67	4.96	5.25	5.54
38–41	FEV_1	3.20	3.42	3.63	3.85	4.06	4.28	4.49
42–45	FVC	3.71	3.99	4.28	4.57	4.84	5.15	5.43
42–45	FEV_1	3.09	3.30	3.52	3.73	3.95	4.16	4.38
46–49	FVC	3.60	3.89	4.18	4.47	4.75	5.04	5.33
46–49	FEV_1	2.97	3.18	3.40	3.61	3.83	4.04	4.26
50–53	FVC	3.50	3.79	4.07	4.36	4.65	4.94	5.23
50–53	FEV_1	2.85	3.07	3.28	3.50	3.71	3.93	4.14
54–57	FVC	3039	3.68	3.97	4.26	4.55	4.83	5.12
54–57	FEV_1	2.74	2.95	3.17	3.38	3.60	3.81	4.03
58–61	FVC	3.29	3058	3.87	4.15	4.44	4.73	5.02
58–61	FEV_1	2.62	2.84	3.05	3.27	3.48	3.70	3.91
62–65	FVC	3.19	3.47	3.76	4.05	4.34	4.63	4.91
62–65	FEV_1	2.51	2.72	2.94	3.15	3.37	3.58	3.80
66–69	FVC	3.08	3.37	3.66	3.95	4.23	4.52	4.81
66–69	FEV_1	2.39	2.60	2.82	3.03	3.25	3.46	3.68

For men over 70 years, predicted values are less well established but can be calculated from the equations below (height in cm; age in years):

$FVC = (0.0576 \times \text{height}) - (0.026 \times \text{age}) - 4.34$ (SD: ± 0.61 L)

$FEV_1 = (0.043 \times \text{height}) - (0.029 \times \text{age}) - 2.49$ (SD: ± 0.51 L)

Female

Age (years)		4'11" 150 cm	5'1" 155 cm	5'3" 160 cm	5'5" 165 cm	5'7" 170 cm	5'9" 175 cm	5'11" 180 cm
38–41	FVC	2.96	2.91	3.13	3.35	3.58	3.80	4.02
38–41	FEV_1	2.30	2.50	2.70	2.89	3.09	3.29	3.49
42–45	FVC	2.59	2.81	3.03	3.25	3.47	3.69	3.91
42–45	FEV_1	2.20	2.40	2.60	2.79	2.99	3.19	3.39
46–49	FVC	2.48	2.70	2.92	3.15	3.37	3.59	3.81
46–49	FEV_1	2.10	2.30	2.50	2.69	2.89	3.09	3.29
50–53	FVC	2.38	2.60	2.82	3.04	3.26	3.48	3.71
50–53	FEV_1	2.00	2.20	2.40	2.59	2.79	2.99	3.19
54–57	FVC	2.27	2.49	2.72	2.94	3.16	3.38	3.60
54–57	FEV_1	1.90	2.10	2.30	2.49	2.69	2.89	3.09
58–61	FVC	2.17	2.39	2.61	2.83	3.06	3.28	3.50
58–61	FEV_1	1.80	2.00	2.20	2.39	2.59	2.79	2.99
62–65	FVC	2.07	2.29	2.51	2.73	2.95	3.17	3.39
62–65	FEV_1	1.70	1.90	2.10	2.29	2.49	2.69	2.89
66–69	FVC	1.96	2.18	2.40	2.63	2.85	3.07	3.29
66–69	FEV_1	1.60	1.80	2.00	2.19	2.39	2.59	2.79

For women over 70 years, predicted values are less well established but can be calculated from the equations below (height in cm; age in years):

$$FVC = (0.0443 \times \text{height}) - (0.026 \times \text{age}) - 2.89 \text{ (SD: } \pm 0.43 \text{ L)}$$

$$FEV_1 = (0.0395 \times \text{height}) - (0.025 \times \text{age}) - 2.60 \text{ (SD: } \pm 0.38 \text{ L)}$$

Reference: Chronic Obstructive Pulmonary Disease. (2004) National clinical guideline for management of chronic obstructive pulmonary disease in adults in primary and secondary care. *Thorax* **59**, (Supplement 1), 1–232.

Antenatal care: routine care for the healthy pregnant woman

- The needs of each pregnant woman should be reassessed at each appointment throughout pregnancy
- At each appointment, women should be given information with an opportunity to discuss issues and ask questions
- Women should usually carry their own case notes
- Women should be informed of the results of all tests
- Verbal information should be supported by classes and written information that is evidence-based
- Identify women who may need additional care (refer to full NICE guidance for list)

At the initial appointment

- Give information on diet and lifestyle, pregnancy care services, maternity benefits, screening tests
- Inform about the benefits of folic acid supplementation
- Offer screening tests – the purpose of each test should be understood before they are undertaken. The right of a woman to accept or decline a test should be made clear
- Support women who smoke by offering antismoking interventions

Prior to 16 weeks' gestation

- Blood tests: blood group, Rhesus status, red cell antibodies, Hb, hepatits B, HIV, rubella susceptibility, syphilis serology
- Urine test for bacteriuria
- Ultrasound scan to determine gestational age
- Down's syndrome screening: nuchal translucency at 11–14 weeks, serum screening at 14–20 weeks

18–20 weeks' gestation onwards

- Ultrasound scan for detection of structural anomalies

At regular intervals (interval depends on parity of woman and fetal and maternal health)

- Review, discuss and record all results of screening tests undertaken
- Measure blood pressure
- Test urine for proteinuria
- Measure symphysis–fundal height (SFH)

In addition, at 28 weeks' gestation

- Offer repeat screening for anaemia and atypical red cell antibodies
- Offer anti-D if Rhesus negative

In addition, at 36 weeks' gestation

- Check presentation. Offer elective caesarean section if breech.

In addition, at 41 weeks' gestation

- Offer membrane sweep
- Offer induction after 41 weeks

Reference: http://www.nice.org.uk/nicemedia/pdf/ANC_FINAL_Algorithm.pdf

PATIENT HEALTH QUESTIONNAIRE (PHQ-9)

NAME:_____ DATE:_____

Over the last *2 weeks,* how often have you been
bothered by any of the following problems?
(use "✓" to indicate your answer)

	Not at all	Several days	More than half the days	Nearly every day
1. Little interest or pleasure in doing things	0	1	2	3
2. Feeling down, depressed, or hopeless	0	1	2	3
3. Trouble falling or staying asleep, or sleeping too much	0	1	2	3
4. Feeling tired or having little energy	0	1	2	3
5. Poor appetite or overeating	0	1	2	3
6. Feeling bad about yourself—or that you are a failure or have let yourself or your family down	0	1	2	3
7. Trouble concentrating on things, such as reading the newspaper or watching television	0	1	2	3
8. Moving or speaking so slowly that other people could have noticed. Or the opposite — being so figety or restless that you have been moving around a lot more than usual	0	1	2	3
9. Thoughts that you would be better off dead, or of hurting yourself	0	1	2	3

add columns [_____] + [_____] + [_____]

(Healthcare professional: For interpretation of TOTAL, TOTAL: [_____]
please refer to accompanying scoring card).

10. If you checked off *any problems,* how *difficult* have these problems made it for you to do your work, take care of things at home, or get along with other people?	Not difficult at all	_____
	Somewhat difficult	_____
	Very difficult	_____
	Extremely difficult	_____

Figure 15 Patient Health Questionnaire (PHQ-9). Copyright © Pfizer Inc. All rights reserved. Reproduced with permission.

PHQ-9 Patient Depression Questionnaire
For initial diagnosis:

1 Patient completes PHQ-9 Quick Depression Assessment.

2 If there are at least 4 √s in the shaded section (including Questions #1 and #2), consider a depressive disorder. Add score to determine severity.

Consider Major Depressive Disorder

If there are at least 5 √s in the shaded section (one of which corresponds to Question #1 or #2)

Consider Other Depressive Disorder

If there are 2–4 √s in the shaded section (one of which corresponds to Question #1 or #2)

Note: Since the questionnaire relies on patient self-report, all responses should be verified by the clinician, and a definitive diagnosis is made on clinical grounds taking into account how well the patient understood the questionnaire, as well as other relevant information from the patient.

Diagnoses of Major Depressive Disorder or Other Depressive Disorder also require impairment of social, occupational, or other important areas of functioning (Question #10) and ruling out normal bereavement, a history of a Manic Episode (Bipolar Disorder), and a physical disorder, medication, or other drug as the biological cause of the depressive symptoms.

To monitor severity over time for newly diagnosed patients or patients in current treatment for depression

1 Patients may complete questionnaires at baseline and at regular intervals (e.g., every 2 weeks) at home and bring them in at their next appointment for scoring or they may complete the questionnaire during each scheduled appointment.

2 Add up √s by column. For every √: Several days = 1 More than half the days = 2 Nearly every day = 3

3 Add together column scores to get a TOTAL score.

4 Refer to the accompanying **PHQ-9 Scoring Box** to interpret the TOTAL score.

5 Results may be included in patient files to assist you in setting up a treatment goal, determining degree of response, as well as guiding treatment intervention.

Scoring: add up all checked boxes on PHQ-9

For every √ Not at all, 0; Several days, 1; More than half the days, 2; Nearly every day, 3.

Interpretation of total score

Total score	Depression severity
1–4	Minimal depression
5–9	Mild depression
10–14	Moderate depression
15–19	Moderately severe depression
20–27	Severe depression

Index of cases by diagnosis

Index

Printed and bound by CPI Group (UK) Ltd, Croydon, CR0 4YY